Interventional Pancreaticobiliary Endoscopy

Editor

TODD H. BARON

GASTROINTESTINAL ENDOSCOPY CLINICS OF NORTH AMERICA

www.giendo.theclinics.com

Consulting Editor
ASHLEY L. FAULX

July 2024 • Volume 34 • Number 3

ELSEVIER

1600 John F. Kennedy Boulevard • Suite 1800 • Philadelphia, Pennsylvania, 19103-2899

http://www.theclinics.com

GASTROINTESTINAL ENDOSCOPY CLINICS OF NORTH AMERICA Volume 34, Number 3
July 2024 ISSN 1052-5157, ISBN-13: 978-0-443-12949-0

Editor: Kerry Holland
Developmental Editor: Malvika Shah

Gastrointestinal Endoscopy Clinics of North America (ISSN 1052-5157) is published quarterly by Elsevier Inc., 360 Park Avenue South, New York, NY 10010-1710. Months of issue are January, April, July, and October. Business and Editorial Offices: 1600 John F. Kennedy Blvd., Suite 1800, Philadelphia, PA, 19103-2899. Periodicals postage paid at New York, NY and additional mailing offices. Subscription prices are $392.00 per year for US individuals, $100.00 per year for US and Canadian students/residents, $432.00 per year for Canadian individuals, $516.00 per year for international individuals, and $245.00 per year for international students/residents. For institutional access pricing please contact Customer Service via the contact information below. To receive student/resident rate, orders must be accompanied by name of affiliated institution, date of term, and the signature of program/residency coordinator on institution letterhead. Orders will be billed at individual rate until proof of status is received. Foreign air speed delivery is included in all Clinics subscription prices. All prices are subject to change without notice. **POSTMASTER:** Send address change to Gastrointestinal Endoscopy Clinics of North America, Elsevier Health Sciences Division, Subscription Customer Service, 3251 Riverport Lane, Maryland Heights, MO 63043. **Customer Service: 1-800-654-2452 (US). From outside the United States, call 1-314-447-8871. Fax: 1-314-447-8029. E-mail: JournalsCustomerService-usa@elsevier.com (for print support) or JournalsOnlineSupport-usa@elsevier.com (for online support).**

Reprints. For copies of 100 or more, of articles in this publication, please contact the Commercial Reprints Department, Elsevier Inc., 360 Park Avenue South, New York, NY 10010-1710. Tel. 212-633-3874; Fax: 212-633-3820; E-mail: reprints@elsevier.com.

Gastrointestinal Endoscopy Clinics of North America is covered in Excerpta Medica, MEDLINE/PubMed (Index Medicus), and MEDLINE/MEDLARS.

Contributors

CONSULTING EDITOR

ASHLEY L. FAULX, MD, MASGE, FACG
Professor of Medicine, Case Western Reserve University School of Medicine, University Hospitals Cleveland Medical Center, Louis Stokes Veterans Affairs Medical Center, Cleveland, Ohio, USA

EDITOR

TODD H. BARON, MD
Professor of Medicine, Director of Therapeutic Endoscopy, Division of Gastroenterology and Hepatology, University of North Carolina, Chapel Hill, North Carolina, USA

AUTHORS

TODD H. BARON, MD
Professor of Medicine, Director of Therapeutic Endoscopy, Division of Gastroenterology and Hepatology, University of North Carolina, Chapel Hill, North Carolina, USA

ALIANA BOFILL-GARCIA, MD
Instructor in Medicine, Department of Gastroenterology and Hepatology, Mayo Clinic Rochester, Rochester, Minnesota, USA

NICHOLAS G. BROWN, MD
Assistant Professor of Medicine, Weill Cornell Medicine, NewYork-Presbyterian/Brooklyn Methodist Hospital, Brooklyn; Columbia University Irving Medical Center, New York, New York, USA

ANDREW CANAKIS, DO
Fellow, Division of Gastroenterology and Hepatology, University of Maryland Medical Center, Baltimore, Maryland, USA

SHANNON MELISSA CHAN, MBChB, FRCSEd, FHKAM (Surgery)
Assistant Professor, Department of Surgery, Prince of Wales Hospital, The Chinese University of Hong Kong, Shatin, Hong Kong, China

HYUNG KU CHON, MD, PhD
Professor, Department of Internal Medicine, Division of Biliopancreas, Wonkwang University Medical School and Hospital, Institution of Wonkwang Medical Science, Iksan, Republic of Korea

KHALED ELFERT, MD
Internal Medicine Resident, St. Barnabas Hospital Health System, City College of New York, CUNY School of Medicine, Bronx, New York, USA

YURI HANADA, MD
Assistant Professor, University of Minnesota Medical School, Division of
Gastroenterology, Hennepin Healthcare, Minneapolis, Minnesota, USA

MARK HANSCOM, MD
Assistant Professor of Medicine, Division of Gastroenterology and Hepatology, Weill
Cornell Medicine, New York, New York, USA

MICHEL KAHALEH, MD
Clinical Director, Department of Gastroenterology, Robert Wood Johnson University
Hospital, New Brunswick, New Jersey, USA

RICHARD A. KOZAREK, MD
Clinical Researcher, Division of Gastroenterology and Hepatology, Center for Digestive
Health, Center for Interventional Immunology, Benaroya Research Institute, Virginia
Mason Franciscan Health, Seattle, Washington, USA

ARJUN KUNDRA, MD
Clinical Instructor, Department of Gastroenterology and Hepatology, University of
Virginia, Charlottesville, Virginia, USA

RYAN LAW, DO
Associate Professor of Medicine, Division of Gastroenterology and Hepatology, Mayo
Clinic Rochester, Rochester, Minnesota, USA

CAMILLE LUPIANEZ-MERLY, MD
Research Fellow, Department of Gastroenterology and Hepatology, Mayo Clinic
Rochester, Rochester, Minnesota, USA

JENNIFER L. MARANKI, MD, MSc, FASGE
Professor of Medicine, Division of Gastroenterology and Hepatology, Penn State College
of Medicine, Penn State Health, Hershey, Pennsylvania, USA

MATTHEW T. MOYER, MD, MS, FASGE
Professor, Department of Medicine, Division of Gastroenterology and Hepatology,
Penn State College of Medicine, Penn State Cancer Institute, Penn State Milton
S. Hershey Medical Center, Hershey, Pennsylvania, USA

HADIE RAZJOUYAN, MD
Associate Professor of Medicine, Division of Gastroenterology and Hepatology,
Penn State College of Medicine, Penn State Health, Hershey, Pennsylvania,
USA

AMRITA SETHI, MD
Professor of Medicine, Division of Digestive and Liver Disease, Columbia University Irving
Medical Center, New York, New York, USA

GULSEREN SEVEN, MD
Professor, Division of Gastroenterology, Bezmialem Foundation University, Bezmialem
Vakif University School of Medicine, Istanbul, Turkey

RAJ J. SHAH, MD, MASGE, AGAF, FACG
Professor, Medicine-Gastroenterology, Division of Gastroenterology and Hepatology,
University of Colorado School of Medicine, Director, Pancreas and Biliary Endoscopy,
Pancreas & Biliary Multidisciplinary Clinic, University of Colorado Anschutz Medical
Campus, Aurora, Colorado, USA

VANESSA M. SHAMI, MD
Chief of Interventional Gastroenterology, Professor, Department of Medicine, University of Virginia, Charlottesville, Virginia, USA

DANIEL S. STRAND, MD
Associate Professor of Medicine, Department of Gastroenterology, University of Virginia, Charlottesville, Virginia, USA

ANTHONY YUEN BUN TEOH, MBChB, FRCSEd, FHKAM (Surgery)
Professor, Department of Surgery, Prince of Wales Hospital, The Chinese University of Hong Kong, Shatin, Hong Kong, China

JUDY A. TRIEU, MD, MPH
Assistant Professor of Medicine, Division of Gastroenterology, Washington University in St. Louis, St Louis, Missouri, USA

AMY TYBERG, MD, FACG, FASGE
Advanced Endoscopist, Hackensack University Medical Center, Hackensack Meridian Medical Group, Hackensack, New Jersey, USA

Contents

 Video content accompanies this article at http://www.giendo.
theclinics.com.

With the introduction of endoscopic retrograde cholangiopancreatography and linear endoscopic ultrasound, interventional pancreaticobiliary (PB) endoscopy has had an enormous impact in the management of pancreatic and biliary diseases. Continuous efforts to improve various devices and techniques have revolutionized these treatment modalities as viable alternatives to surgery. In recent years, trends toward combining endoscopic techniques with other modalities, such as laparoscopic and radiological interventions, for complex PB diseases have emerged using a multidisciplinary approach. Ongoing research and clinical experience will lead to refinements in interventional PB endoscopic techniques and subsequently improve outcomes and reduce complication rates.

Pancreatic duct (PD) leaks are a common complication of acute and chronic pancreatitis, trauma to the pancreas, and pancreatic surgery. Diagnosis of PD leaks and fistulas is often made with contrast-enhanced pancreatic protocol computed tomography or magnetic resonance imaging with MRCP. Endoscopic retrograde pancreatography with pancreatic duct stenting in appropriately selected patients is often an effective treatment, helps to avoid surgery, and is considered first-line therapy in cases that fail conservative management.

 Video content accompanies this article at http://www.giendo.
theclinics.com.

Per-oral pancreatoscopy (POP) is a pancreas-preserving modality that allows for targeted pancreatic duct interventions, particularly in cases where standard techniques fail. POP specifically has an emerging role in the diagnosis, risk stratification, and disease extent determination of main

endoscopic transpapillary gallbladder drainage for patients suffering from acute calculous cholecystitis who are at high risk for surgery. Multiple cohorts, meta-analyses, and a randomized controlled trial have shown that EUS-GBD has lower rates of recurrent cholecystitis and unplanned reinterventions, while achieving similar technical and clinical success rates than transpapillary cystic duct stenting. The essential steps, precautions in performing EUS-GBD and long-term management will be discussed in this article.

Endoscopic Ultrasound-Guided Ablation of Pancreatic Mucinous Cysts

Matthew T. Moyer and Andrew Canakis

Endoscopic ultrasound (EUS) has rapidly evolved from a diagnostic to a therapeutic tool with applications for various pancreaticobiliary diseases. As part of this evolution, EUS-guided chemoablation for neoplastic pancreatic cysts is developing as a minimally invasive treatment option for appropriately selected mucinous cysts, which can spare patients major resective surgery and may reduce progression to pancreatic cancer. Chemotherapeutic cyst ablation has demonstrated encouraging complete resolution rates, while an alcohol-free chemoablation protocol has demonstrated a significant decrease in adverse events without a compromise to complete ablation rates when compared with previous alcohol-based protocols. Most pancreatic cysts are small, low risk, and best managed by surveillance per accepted guidelines. Cysts with features suggestive of overt malignancy are best discussed by a multidisciplinary committee, and surgery is considered if appropriate. However, for patients in the middle ground with cysts that are structurally suitable for chemoablation, alcohol-free chemoablation has been shown to allow effective, safe, and durable results especially for those who are not ideal operative candidates. EUS-guided alcohol-free chemoablation is promising and continues to evolve; however, as a relatively novel treatment option it has areas of uncertainty that will require further investigation and development.

Endoscopic Drainage of Pancreatic Fluid Collections

Nicholas G. Brown and Amrita Sethi

 Video content accompanies this article at http://www.giendo. theclinics.com

Pancreatic fluid collections (PFCs) are commonly encountered complications of acute and chronic pancreatitis. With the advancement of endoscopic ultrasound (EUS) techniques and devices, EUS-directed transmural drainage of symptomatic or infected PFCs has become the standard of care. Traditionally, plastic stents have been used for drainage, although lumen-apposing metal stents (LAMSs) are now favored by most endoscopists due to ease of use and reduced procedure time. While safety has been repeatedly demonstrated, follow-up care for these patients is critical as delayed adverse events of indwelling drains are known to occur.

GASTROINTESTINAL ENDOSCOPY CLINICS OF NORTH AMERICA

SERIES OF RELATED INTEREST

Gastroenterology Clinics
(www.gastro.theclinics.com)
Clinics in Liver Disease
(www.liver.theclinics.com)

THE CLINICS ARE AVAILABLE ONLINE!
Access your subscription at:
www.theclinics.com

Foreword

The Ever-Expanding Role of Endoscopy in Pancreaticobiliary Disease

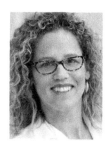

Ashley L. Faulx, MD, MASGE, FACG
Consulting Editor

This issue focuses on Interventional Pancreaticobiliary Endoscopy lead by Guest Editor Dr Todd Baron, a world-renowned expert in interventional endoscopy and a pioneer in novel interventional endoscopy techniques over the past three decades. Dr Baron has assembled leaders in the field of interventional endoscopy to discuss a wide range of techniques, from imaging to interventions to managing challenging pancreatic and biliary diseases in addition to the challenges presented to the endoscopist in patients with altered anatomy. It is an exciting time for therapeutic endoscopists, as we can offer our patients endoscopic options for therapy, previously treated with surgery, and its associated morbidity. New techniques also enable the interventionalist to endoscopically evaluate the pancreas and bile duct to perhaps obviate surgical intervention at all. The field continues to evolve rapidly, and this issue represents the state-of-the-art in pancreaticobiliary endoscopy in 2024.

Ashley L. Faulx, MD, MASGE, FACG
Case Western Reserve University
School of Medicine
UH Cleveland Medical Center
Louis Stokes VAMC
11100 Euclid Avenue, Wearn 2nd Floor
Cleveland, OH 44106, USA

E-mail address:
Ashley.faulx@uhhospitals.org

Gastrointest Endoscopy Clin N Am 34 (2024) xiii
https://doi.org/10.1016/j.giec.2024.03.002
1052-5157/24/© 2024 Elsevier Inc. All rights reserved.

Preface

Pancreaticobiliary Endoscopy: Look How Far We've Come

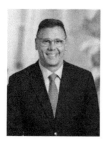

Todd H. Baron, MD
Editor

Having finished my endoscopy training more than 30 years ago, I have witnessed an amazing evolution in therapeutic endoscopy, particularly in pancreaticobiliary endoscopy as covered in this issue of *Gastrointestinal Endoscopy Clinics of North America*. Not to be outdone, my mentor, Richard A. Kozarek, has witnessed even more as a major contributor and detailed the history of pancreaticobiliary endoscopy in his article with Chon entitled "History of the Interventional Pancreaticobiliary Endoscopy." Indeed, his early work and that of others laid the foundation of what we do today.

To think that the diseases discussed in this issue were once only treatable with limited medical options and open surgery seems unfathomable now. In this issue of *Gastrointestinal Endoscopy Clinics of North America*, we have assembled experts to provide insight into the latest endoscopic therapies for pancreaticobiliary diseases.

Pancreatic duct leaks and fistulae, also once only treatable with medications and morbid surgical procedures, have become relatively easily managed with endoscopic therapy as discussed in the article in this issue, "Endoscopic Retrograde Cholangiopancreatography for Management of Pancreatic Duct Leaks and Fistula" by Razjouyan and Maranki. Similarly, pain in the setting of chronic pancreatitis can be managed endoscopically by relief of pancreatic ductal obstruction and endoscopic ultrasound (EUS)-guided celiac injection as discussed in "Pancreatoscopy-Guided Endotherapies for Pancreatic Diseases" by Hanada and Shah, "Endoscopic Management of Pain Due to Chronic Pancreatitis" by Kundra, Strand and Shami, and "Endoscopic Retrograde Cholangiopancreatography for Management of Chronic Pancreatitis" by Bofill-Garcia and Lupianez-Merly.

Pancreatoscopy, once performed using fragile "baby" endoscopes passed via large-caliber "mother scopes," has evolved to single-operator digital imaging endoscopes that pass through standard therapeutic channel duodenoscopes and allow

https://doi.org/10.1016/j.giec.2024.03.001

the endoscopist to detect intraductal disease, such as intrapancreatic mucinous neoplasia and malignancy, and to provide therapies, including electrohydraulic lithotripsy and laser therapies, for pancreatic duct calculi and strictures as discussed in the articles by Hanada and Shah, Kundra, Strand and Shami, and Bofill-Garcia, Lupianez-Merly.

While endoscopic retrograde cholangiopancreatography remains the main endoscopic modality for the nonoperative management of pancreaticobiliary disease, EUS has rapidly gained ground. EUS remains useful not only in its diagnostic capabilities but also as a therapeutic modality allowing creation of enteric anastomoses that allow access to the pancreaticobiliary system in patients with surgically altered anatomy, and by creation of anastomoses directly from the bile duct or pancreas to the gastrointestinal lumen ("Approaches to Pancreaticobiliary Endoscopy in Roux-en-Y Gastric Bypass Anatomy" by Elfert and Kahaleh, "Endoscopic Ultrasound Guided Biliary Drainage (EUS-BD)" by Canakis and Tyberg, "Endoscopic Ultrasound-Guided Pancreatic Duct Drainage", Trieu et al, and "Transenteric ERCP in Non-Roux-en-Y Surgically Altered Anatomy", Hanscom and Law. Symptomatic gallbladder disease, once only treatable with surgery or percutaneous approaches, can now be managed endoscopically via EUS-guided transmural drainage using a device FDA-approved for cholecystitis in poor operative candidates as discussed in "Endoscopic Ultrasonography-Guided Gallbladder Drainage" by Teoh and Chan. Ablative therapies in the pancreas are also emerging as discussed in "EUS-Guided Ablation of Pancreatic Mucinous Cysts" by Moyer and Canakis. Finally, transmural drainage of pancreatic fluid collections has become standard of care, and the use of a variety of plastic and metal stents as tailored to their disease is discussed in "Endoscopic Drainage of Pancreatic Fluid Collections" by Brown and Sethi. In all, this issue represents the culmination of more than 40 years of peroral flexible endoscopy and is intended to enlighten the reader as to how these efforts have translated into clinical care.

Todd H. Baron, MD
Division of Gastroenterology and Hepatology
University of North Carolina
Chapel Hill, NC, USA

E-mail address:
todd_baron@med.unc.edu

History of the Interventional Pancreaticobiliary Endoscopy

Hyung Ku Chon, MD, PhD[a,b], Richard A. Kozarek, MD[c,d],*

KEYWORDS

- Endoscopic retrograde cholangiopancreatography
- Endoscopic ultrasound-guided intervention • Bile duct stone
- Endoscopic gallbladder drainage • Bile duct stricture • Bile duct leak
- Pancreatic pseudocyst • Walled-off necrosis

KEY POINTS

- Endoscopic retrograde cholangiopancreatography and linear endoscopic ultrasound (EUS) play complementary roles and their development has contributed to the advancement of interventional pancreaticobiliary endoscopy.
- The development of endoscopic stenting allows for the alleviation of obstructions in pancreatic or bile ducts.
- Management of pancreaticobiliary diseases has significantly improved due to the introduction of minimally invasive EUS-guided intervention.
- Endoscopic local tumor therapy may lead to improved symptom control, quality of life, and survival rates. However, further research is required.

 Video content accompanies this article at http://www.giendo.theclinics.com.

INTRODUCTION

In the mid-1970s and 1980s, the development of therapeutic endoscopic retrograde cholangiopancreatography (ERCP) techniques laid the foundation for interventional pancreaticobiliary (PB) endoscopy.[1] In the 1990s, with advancements in ERCP

---

[a] Division of Biliopancreas, Department of Internal Medicine, Wonkwang University Medical School, and Hospital, Iksan, Republic of Korea; [b] Institution of Wonkwang Medical Science, Iksan, Republic of Korea; [c] Division of Gastroenterology and Hepatology, Center for Digestive Health, Virginia Mason Franciscan Health, 1100 Ninth Avenue, Seattle, WA 98101, USA; [d] Center for Interventional Immunology, Benaroya Research Institute, Virginia Mason Franciscan Health, 1201 Ninth Avenue, Seattle, WA 98101, USA
* Corresponding author. Division of Gastroenterology and Hepatology, Center for Digestive Health, Virginia Mason Franciscan Health, 1100 Ninth Avenue, Seattle, WA 98101.
E-mail address: richard.kozarek@virginiamason.org

Gastrointest Endoscopy Clin N Am 34 (2024) 383–403
https://doi.org/10.1016/j.giec.2023.12.001
1052-5157/24/© 2023 Elsevier Inc. All rights reserved.
giendo.theclinics.com

techniques and the development of linear endoscopic ultrasound (EUS), interventional PB endoscopy became more specialized and widespread.[1,2] Moreover, with the application of computed tomography (CT) and MRI, PB endoscopy has evolved toward therapeutic interventions rather than for solely diagnostic purposes. Device and accessory innovations in conjunction with ongoing research have demonstrated that PB endoscopy can be an effective alternative to surgery for many PB disorders. This article discusses the historic developments in interventional PB endoscopy.

BILE DUCT STONES

The development of endoscopic sphincterotomy (EST) with ERCP revolutionized bile duct stone treatment. In 1968, McCune performed the first successful ERCP and in 1974, Classen and colleagues and Kawai and colleagues performed pioneering EST for the management of biliary tract diseases (**Table 1**).[3–5] Since the 1980s, various instruments have been developed for stone removal and fragmentation. This has led to a high success rate of endoscopic bile duct stone removal approximating 85% to 90% and lower adverse event (AE) rates, shorter hospital stays, and lower mortality rate than surgery.[6,7] However, complete stone removal may be difficult in approximately 10% to 15% of cases. For such cases, alternative approaches, such as mechanical lithotripsy (ML), intraductal electrohydraulic lithotripsy (EHL), laser lithotripsy (LL), endoscopic papillary large-balloon dilation (EPLBD), and temporary biliary stenting, may be used.

Riemann and colleagues first described ML in 1982, with a success rate of 79% to 92% for stones that could not be removed using conventional methods.[8–10] EHL was first reported in 1977 by Koch and colleagues.[11] In 1986, a neodymium-doped yttrium aluminum garnet laser was used to fracture bile duct stones.[12] With advancements in these technologies, EHL and LL have become widely used to treat bile duct stones when other methods fail with a meta-analysis demonstrating a clearance rate of 88% using digital cholangioscopy (95% confidence interval [CI], 85%–91%; **Fig. 1**, Video 1).[13,14]

In 2003, Ersoz and colleagues reported on the combination of EST and EPLBD using 12 to 20-mm balloon catheters.[15] This approach is a safe and effective for patients with difficult bile duct stones and in patients with large common bile duct (CBD) stones, complete clearance has been reported in 95% to 100% with AEs occurring in 0% to 16%.[16–19]

ENDOSCOPIC TREATMENT OF BENIGN AND MALIGNANT BILIARY STRICTURES

Initial endoscopic treatment of biliary strictures involved mechanical dilation, endoscopic nasobiliary drainage (ENBD), and plastic stent (PS) placement alone or in combination. Balloon dilation of biliary strictures was first developed in the late 1970s.[20] There has been modest refinement of balloon catheters but dilation alone is seldom used and is used in conjunction with other methods.[21]

ENBD was first reported by Nagai and colleagues in 1976, and Wurbs and colleagues described the use of a specialized long radiopaque biliary tube in 1980.[22,23] In 1979, Soehendra and colleagues first described endoscopic transpapillary drainage using a 7-Fr pigtail PS via ERCP for malignant biliary obstruction.[24]

The subsequent development of self-expandable metallic stents (SEMSs) significantly improved the ease of deployment and prolonged patency of biliary stents compared with 10Fr PSs.[25,26] In 1989, the first endoscopic biliary SEMS was reported in 33 patients with malignant extrahepatic bile duct strictures with a 100% technical success rate and 96.6% clinical success rate (32 out of 33).[25]

Table 1
Evolution of interventional endoscopy for biliary disease

	Author, Year
Bile duct stone	
EST and extraction of stones	Classen et al,[4] 1974; Kawai et al,[5] 1974
Mechanical lithotripter for fracturing CBD stones	Riemann et al,[8] 1982
EHL for fragmentation of large CBD stone	Koch et al,[11] 1977
LL of CBD stones	Lux et al,[12] 1986
Endoscopic papillary large balloon dilation with EST for difficult bile duct stone	Ersoz el al,[15] 2003
Single operator cholangioscopy-directed biliary stone therapy	Chen et al,[13] 2011
Biliary stricture	
Biliary stricture dilatation using a balloon catheter	Burhenne et al,[20] 1980
Endoscopic naso-biliary drainage	Nagai et al,[22] 1976
PS placement using a 7Fr pigtail	Soehendra et al,[24] 1979
Endoscopic placement of SEMS for biliary strictures	Huibregtse et al,[25] 1989
Survival benefit of bilateral drainage for MHBO, compared with unilateral drainage	Chang et al,[40] 1998
EUS-CDS for biliary drainage in patient with pancreatic cancer after failed ERCP	Giovannini et al,[42] 2001
EUS-HGS as a palliative treatment in a patient with metastatic biliary obstruction	Giovannini et al,[45] 2003
Antegrade stenting with EUS-HDS in patients with isolated right hepatic duct obstruction	Park et al,[46] 2013
EUS-RV drainage of obstructed biliary and pancreatic ducts	Mallery et al,[44] 2004
Acute cholecystitis	
Transpapillary GB catheter insertion	Foerster et al,[48] 1988
Endoscopic naso-GB drain	Feretis et al,[50] 1990
EUS-GBD with a 7Fr double pigtail stent	Baron et al,[52] 2007
EUS-GBD with a modified covered SEMS	Jang et al,[53] 2011
EUS-GBD with LAMSs	Itoi et al,[54] 2012
Bile leak	
EST and PS replacement for cholecystectomy related bile leak	Kozarek et al,[61] 1994
Covered SEMS for closure of complex biliary leaks	Baron et al,[62] 2006

Abbreviations: CBD, common bile duct; EST, endoscopic sphincterotomy; EUS, endoscopic ultrasound; GB, gallbladder; GBD, gallbladder drainage; MHBO, malignant hilar biliary obstruction; SBS, stent by stent; SEMS, Self-expandable metal stent; SIS, stent in stent.

Placement of multiple PS or a single, fully covered SEMS (FCSEMS) is now used for the treatment of benign biliary strictures (BBSs).[27–29] The larger diameter FCSEMS provide prolonged stent patency than PS and requires fewer procedures than serial dilatation or multiplastic stenting with low AE rates and high cost-effectiveness, although not clearly superior to multiplastic stenting for BBSs.[27,30–34]

For malignant distal biliary obstruction ERCP with SEMS placement is now the treatment of choice, although recent meta-analyses suggest no significant difference in stent patency or AEs between covered and uncovered SEMSs (**Fig. 2**).[35–39]

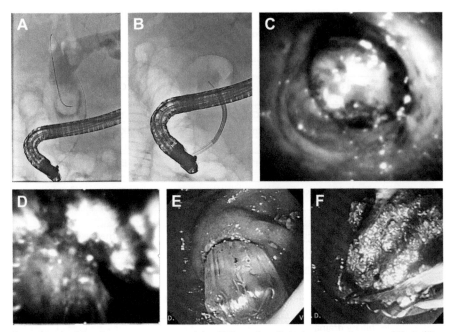

Fig. 1. Large bile duct stone removed by EHL under digital cholangioscopy. (*A*) A filing defect measuring approximately 3 cm can be seen along the bile duct on fluoroscopy. (*B–D*) Stone fragmentation using EHL under digital cholangioscopy. (*E, F*) Stone extraction with a basket following endoscopic papillary large balloon dilation.

Endoscopic drainage for patients with malignant hilar biliary obstruction (MHBO) is technically challenging. Chang and colleagues first described the survival benefits of bilateral drainage for MHBO in 1998.[40] One prospective randomized controlled trial (RCT) demonstrated that bilateral SEMS placement was superior to unilateral SEMS placement in terms of the reintervention rate and stent patency, whereas the technical success rate was similar between the 2 groups.[41]

In the 1990s and 2000s, EUS-guided biliary drainage (EUS-BD), which includes EUS-guided choledochoduodenostomy (EUS-CDS), EUS-guided hepaticogastrostomy (EUS-HGS), EUS-guided hepaticoduodenostomy (EUS-HDS), and EUS-guided rendezvous (EUS-RV), expanded the treatment options for malignant biliary obstruction and provided solutions in cases of failed ERCP or inaccessible papilla.[42–44]

In 2001, Giovannini and colleagues first described the use of EUS-CDS for relief of distal MBO in a patient who failed ERCP.[42] FCSEMS with flared ends or lumen-apposing metal stent (LAMS) placement is preferred to prevent the risk of bile leakage (**Fig. 3**). Prospective studies have shown comparable safety and a lower incidence of tumor in-growth in SEMS compared with ERCP using EUS-CDS.

EUS-HGS was first reported in 2003 and has evolved as a modality for relief of MHBO in patients with failed ERCP or surgically altered anatomy (SAA).[45] In 2013, Park and colleagues reported anterograde stenting with HDS.[46]

In 2004, Mallery and colleagues first described the use of EUS-RV after an unsuccessful ERCP.[44] One systematic review reported the technical success rate of EUS-RV to be 86.1% (95% CI, 78.4%–91.3%), with a clinical success rate of 80.8% (95% CI, 64.1%–90.8%) and an AE rate of 14% (95% CI, 10.5%–18.4%).[47]

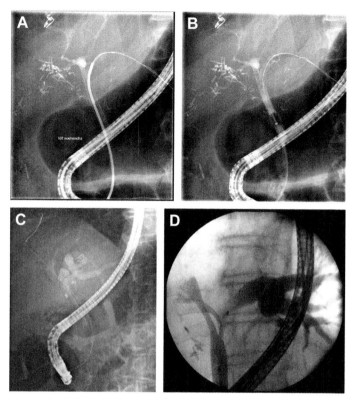

Fig. 2. Various methods for metallic stent placement through ERCP in the treatment of a hilar cholangiocarcinoma. (*A, B*) Stent in stent. (*C*) Side by side. (*D*) Triple stenting. (Fig. 2D was originally published [Kozarek RA. Inflammation and carcinogenesis of the biliary tract: update on endoscopic treatment. Clin Gastroenterol Hepatol. 2009 Nov;7(11 Suppl):S89-94] with permission from Elsevier.)

ENDOSCOPIC GALLBLADDER DRAINAGE

Transpapillary gallbladder (GB) catheter insertion was first described by Foerster and colleagues on 8 autopsy preparations.[48] Initially, used to dissolve stone fragments after extracorporeal shock wave lithotripsy (ESWL) for gallstones, Feretis and colleagues demonstrated treatment of GB empyema using an endoscopic nasoGB drain in 1990.[49,50] Transpapillary GB drainage has a technical success rate of 75% to 96% and a clinical success rate of 86.7% to 100%.[51]

EUS-guided GB drainage (EUS-GBD) for acute cholecystitis was first described by Baron and Topazian in 2007 using a 7-Fr double pigtail stent.[52] Placement of a modified covered SEMS was first used for EUS-GBD in 2011 (Video 2).[53] In 2012, a newly developed LAMS was introduced as a novel tool for EUS-guided transluminal drainage procedures. Itoi and colleagues first described LAMS placement for pancreatic pseudocyst (PP) and GB drainage.[54] A recent systematic review showed statistically significantly higher technical and clinical success rates and lower recurrence rates with EUS-GBD than endoscopic transpapillary GB drainage. Compared with percutaneous cholecystostomy, EUS-GBD showed a significantly lower reintervention rate with similar efficacy and safety.[55]

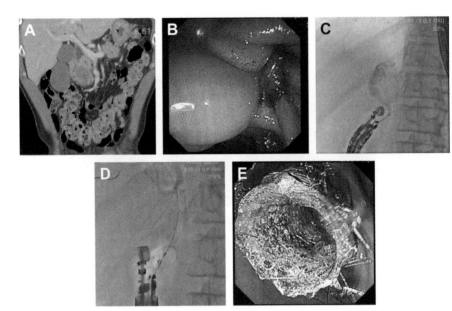

Fig. 3. EUS-guided choledochoduodenostomy for malignant biliary obstruction after failed endoscopic retrograde cholangiopancreatography. (*A*) Abdominal CT showing a 2.5-cm irregular mass located in the pancreatic head, accompanied by bile duct dilatation. (*B*) Endoscopic image showing ampulla deformity caused by invasion of the pancreatic head cancer. (*C*) Fluoroscopy image showing a cholangiogram following the puncture of the dilated bile duct using a 19-G fine needle aspiration needle. (*D*) Fluoroscopy image showing a biflanged fully covered metallic stent placed between the bile duct and duodenum. (*E*) Endoscopic image showing drainage of bile through the stent.

BILE LEAK AND BILE INJURY

Treatment modalities for bile leaks include surgery, percutaneous drainage (PCD), and endoscopic approaches. Surgery-related morbidity (22%–37%) and mortality (3%–18%) is high and often with unsatisfactory outcomes.[56,57] In the late 1980s, case reports demonstrated promising results for ERCP with EST, nasobiliary drainage, PS placement, or a combination for treatment of bile leaks.[58–60]

The widespread adoption of laparoscopic cholecystectomy in the 1990s led to an increase in bile leakage. In a case series by Kozarek and colleagues, of the described 29 patients with biliary injuries who underwent EST and PS placement following laparoscopic or open cholecystectomy, 25 were successfully treated.[61]

FCSEMS placement can be a useful option for managing bile leaks originating from the cystic duct remnant, CBD, or common hepatic duct or in cases of refractory bile leak following PS placement. In 2006, Baron and Poterucha first used partially covered SEMS to close complex bile leaks.[62] Since then, 40 patients were treated for postcholecystectomy bile leaks that did not resolve after PS placement. Patients were treated with either FCSEMS placement (n = 20) or multiple PS insertions (n = 20). FCSEMS placement resulted in a higher rate of bile leak closure (65% vs 100%, *P*=.004).[63]

PANCREATIC PSEUDOCYST AND WALLED-OFF NECROSIS

Peripancreatic fluid collection (PFC) resulting from acute pancreatitis is categorized into acute peripancreatic fluid collection, acute necrotic collection, PP, and walled-off necrosis (WON).[64] Historically, surgery was the primary treatment of PP.[65] In the 1970s and 1980s, PCD emerged as a less-invasive alternative to surgery.[66–68] In 1975, the first endoscopic transgastric needle aspiration was performed in a patient with a 10-cm PP (**Table 2**).[69]

The first description of endoscopic transluminal PP drainage was performed by Kozarek and colleagues using a modified straight-wire sphincterotome through the stomach or duodenum in 4 high-risk surgical patients.[70]

In 1992, Grimm and colleagues first described EUS-guided cystogastrostomy using a 10-Fr pigtail PS without evidence of extraluminal bulging.[71] Four years later, Wiersema and colleagues first described PP drainage guided completely by EUS after a failed endoscopic transluminal approach.[72] Linear EUS allows for precise localization and characterization of PP as well as the identification of any intervening vessels at the puncture site with a higher success rate and lower AE rate than endoscopic transluminal drainage for PP (**Fig. 4**).[73,74]

Surgical necrosectomy was historically the primary treatment of WON. With advancements in endoscopic treatment of PP, the same approach has been used for WON. In 1996, Baron and colleagues first used transluminal drainage for the treatment

Table 2	
Evolution of interventional endoscopy for pancreatic disease	
	Author, Year
Pancreatic fluid collection	
Endoscopic trans-gastric needle aspiration using a 21-gauge needle for 10 cm PP	Rogers et al,[69] 1975
Endoscopic transluminal PP drainage using a modified straight wire sphincterotome	Kozarek et al,[70] 1985
EUS-guided PP drainage	Wiersema,[72] 1996
Endoscopic necrosectomy and lavage for infected WON	Baron et al,[75] 1996
"Step-up" approach showing lower incidence of multiorgan failure	van Santvoort et al,[80] 2010
Pancreatic duct leak with DPDS	
Endoscopic transpapillary therapy for disrupted pancreatic duct	Kozarek et al,[82] 1991
Combination of transpapillary drainage, cystogastrostomy or cystoduodenostomy, or naso-cystic catheter for complete disruption of the main pancreatic duct	Deviere et al,[85] 1995
Pancreatic calculi	
ERCP with basket stone retrieval	Inui et al,[91] 1985
ERCP with pancreatic sphincterotomy, pancreatoscopy with basket stone retrieval, and tran-papillary pancreatic duct stenting	Fuji et al,[92] 1985
ESWL with ERCP	Sauerbruch et al,[93] 1987
EHL using peroral pancreatoscopy with a 10Fr baby endoscope	Howell et al,[100] 1999
Pancreatic duct stricture	
Prospective study showing efficacy of placing multiple PSs	Costamagna et al,[101] 2007
Self-expandable metal stent placement	Eisendrath et al,[103] 1999

Abbreviations: DPDS, disconnected pancreatic duct syndrome; ERCP, endoscopic retrograde cholangiopancreatography; EUS, endoscopic ultrasound; PP, pancreatic pseudocyst.

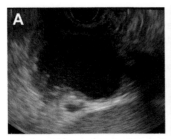 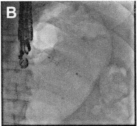 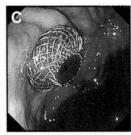

Fig. 4. EUS-guided pancreatic fluid collection drainage using a LAMS for WON. (*A*) EUS image displaying WON with necrotic materials. (*B*) Fluoroscopic image showing the placement of the LAMS between the WON and the stomach. (*C*) Endoscopic image showing pus-like drainage from the LAMS.

of organized pancreatic necrosis (now known as WON).[75] In 2000, Seifert and colleagues described successful treatment of infected WON in 3 patients with direct endoscopic necrosectomy (DEN).[76] Several studies have reported treatment success rates of 75% to 91%, AE rates of 26% to 33%, and mortality rates of 5.8% to 11% using DEN.[77–79]

In 2010, an RCT compared surgical necrosectomy with a "step-up" approach using percutaneous or endoscopic drainage. There was no significant difference in mortality rates but the incidence of multiorgan failure was lower in the "step-up" group and 35% of the patients did not undergo a necrosectomy.[80] In a study comparing DEN with surgical necrosectomy, procedural and postprocedural complications were significantly lower in the DEN group.[81] According to these results, the "step-up" approach has been established as a treatment strategy for infected WON.

PANCREATIC DUCT LEAK

PD leaks were traditionally managed through surgical intervention and often involve complex and invasive procedures. Transpapillary PD stenting with ERCP has been used in the management of PD leaks and fistulas (**Fig. 5**).[82,83] Bridging the leak site through stent placement is crucial for treatment success.[84] However, this treatment is not successful in the setting of complete transection and impossible in the presence of disconnected PD syndrome (DPDS).

In 1995, Deviere and colleagues first described endoscopic transluminal drainage for DPDS.[85] Subsequently, EUS-guided transmural drainage was used to treat patients with DPDS accompanied by a PFC.[86,87] However, in patients with DPDS, recurrence was reported when the PS used for transmural drainage was removed or migrated early.[88,89] In such patients, maintaining the PS has become the standard treatment approach.

PANCREATIC CALCULI

Pancreatic calculi can obstruct the flow of pancreatic juices, leading to an increase in pressure within the PD and capsule distention, resulting in abdominal pain, nausea, vomiting, maldigestion, jaundice, fever, or diabetes. Painful or pancreatitis-exacerbating stones are indications for treatment. Surgical intervention was first reported by Capparelli in 1883 and historically has been the primary treatment approach.[90] A century later, Inui and colleagues first described endoscopic removal

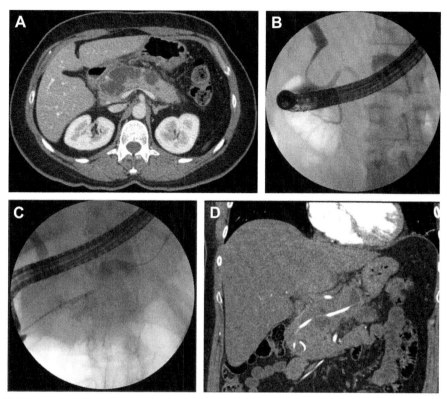

Fig. 5. Transpapillary pancreatic duct stenting for disconnected pancreatic duct syndrome (DPDS). (*A*) Abdominal CT demonstrating fluid collection along the proximal body of pancreas, suggesting possible DPDS. (*B*) Endoscopic retrograde pancreatography showing DPDS. (*C*) Fluoroscopy showing a guidewire passing beyond the disconnected pancreatic duct. (*D*) Abdominal CT showing PS placement for managing DPDS.

of PD stones by pancreatic sphincterotomy and basket retrieval followed by a case series reported by Fuji and colleagues in 1985.[91,92]

In 1987, Sauerbruch and colleagues first reported successful treatment of an obstructing PD stone using ESWL.[93] Since then, many studies have reported the effectiveness of endoscopic treatment in conjunction with ESWL.[94–99] In 1999, Howell and colleagues performed EHL for the treatment of pancreatic calculi using peroral pancreatoscopy with a 10-Fr baby endoscope.[100]

PANCREATIC DUCT STRICTURES

PD strictures are usually a complication of pancreatic calculi, inflammation, or following necrosis around the PD. The primary goal of endoscopic treatment of PD strictures is to alleviate abdominal pain or acute recurrent pancreatitis. Advancements in endoscopic treatment of PD strictures have been similar to those for biliary strictures.

Endoscopic pancreatic sphincterotomy was first described in 1985 by Fuji and colleagues to enhance PD access.[92] In 2007, Costamagna and colleagues described the efficacy of multiplastic stenting for the treatment of benign PD strictures. The dominant stricture of the PD resolved in 18 of the 19 patients (95%) after the removal of multiple stents. During a follow-up period of 38 months, 84% of patients remained without recurrence of pain, whereas 10.5% had PD stricture recurrence.[101] Although no prospective study has directly compared single versus multiple PS placement, multiple PS may reduce the recurrence rate of PD strictures (30% vs 10.5%).[102]

SEMS placement has been used to reduce the number of endoscopic procedures and enhance the effectiveness of treatments for PD strictures. In 1999, partially covered SEMS were used for the treatment of stenotic ducts. However, most patients experienced mucosal hyperplasia, leading to stent occlusion 6 months later.[103] Subsequently, FCSEMSs of various shapes have been developed and treatment success rates have been reported.[104,105]

EUS-guided interventions, which were introduced in 2002 for select patients with PD strictures, is particularly useful when the conventional transpapillary approach fails or in cases of SAA.[106] These interventions involve draining the MPD using a transmural approach or via transpapillary rendezvous. EUS-guided interventions are effective in reducing pain in 60% to 70% of cases but it is technically challenging to perform.

ENDOSCOPIC ULTRASOUND-GUIDED CELIAC PLEXUS BLOCKAGE

Celiac plexus blockage, including celiac plexus neurolysis (CPN) and celiac plexus block (CPB) is an effective method for alleviating pain caused by chronic pancreatitis and pancreatic cancer.[107] CPB involves administration of an anesthetic (bupivacaine) and steroid (triamcinolone) around the celiac plexus, whereas CPN involves the administration of an anesthetic and alcohol. Historically, surgical, CT-guided, or fluoroscopy-guided percutaneous CPN have been performed.

In 1996, Wiersema and colleagues first reported EUS-CPN using a 22-gauge needle by injecting 0.25% bupivacaine and a 98% dehydrated absolute solution to relieve pancreatic cancer pain. Pain scores improved from 79% to 88% among the 30 subjects, although 4 experienced mild AEs, such as transient diarrhea and hypotension, during a median follow-up period of 12 weeks.[108] Since then, prospective studies have confirmed these results.[109]

INTERVENTIONAL PANCREATICOBILIARY ENDOSCOPY FOR SURGICALLY ALTERED ANATOMY

ERCP in patients with SAA can be challenging. In 1975, Katon and colleagues first described ERCP for patients with Billroth II gastrectomy using a forward-viewing gastroscope.[110] In 1988, Gostout and colleagues first reported the use of a pediatric colonoscope for ERCP in patients with Roux-en-Y anastomosis and hepaticojejunostomy.[111]

Following the initial description of double balloon enteroscopy (DBE) for small bowel examination in 2001, ERCP in SAA, particularly Roux-en-Y anastomosis, was revolutionized.[112] In 2008, Monkemuller and colleagues first reported the use of single balloon enteroscopy (SBE) for ERCP in patients with Roux-en-Y anastomosis.[113] Saleem and colleagues demonstrated successful SBE in 39 of 56 procedures following failure of the use of a colonoscope. Therapeutic procedures were successful in 21 of the 23 cases.[114]

Roux-en-Y gastric bypass (RYGB) has been shown to be highly effective in achieving significant and sustained weight loss in patients with obesity. However, rapid weight loss after RYGB can lead to the formation of gallstones. In 1998, Baron and Vicker described creation of a surgical gastrostomy to allow subsequent ERCP for the management of acute recurrent pancreatitis.[115] In 2002, Peters and colleagues

first described laparoscopic transgastric-ERCP for the treatment of benign CBD strictures in a patient who had previously undergone RYGB.[116]

In 2014, Kedia and colleagues described EUS-guided creation of an anastomosis to
the excluded stomach using LAMS to allow ERCP to be performed using a standard
side-viewing endoscope.[117] This method has been reported to not only reduce the
duration (49.8 minutes vs 90.7 minutes, $P<.001$) but also significantly increase the success rate of the procedure compared with ERCP using DBE or SBE (100% vs 60%,
$P<.001$).[118]

ENDOSCOPIC LOCAL TUMOR THERAPY FOR PANCREATIC AND BILIARY NEOPLASMS
Endoscopic Ultrasound-Guided Pancreatic Cyst Ablation

EUS-guided ethanol lavage (EUS-EL) was first described by Gan and colleagues in
2005 (**Table 3**).[119] In a study involving 25 patients with pancreatic cystic neoplasms
(PCNs), a single session of EUS-EL resulted in cyst resolution in 8 patients.

Subsequently, EUS-guided EL with paclitaxel injection was performed in 14 patients
with PCNs.[120] At follow-up, an average of 9 months after the procedure, complete resolution of the PCNs was observed in 11 out of 14 patients, whereas partial resolution
was noted in 2 out of 14 patients. One patient showed no response. AEs included
asymptomatic amylase elevation (6 patients), pancreatitis (1 patient), and abdominal
pain (1 patient).

Endoscopic Ultrasound-Guided Solid Pancreatic Tumor Ablation

EUS-guided tumor ablation is used to treat solid pancreatic tumors, including pancreatic neuroendocrine tumors (PNETs) and solid pseudopapillary tumors (SPTs). In
2006, Jurgensen and colleagues first performed EUS-guided ethanol ablation in an
elderly patient with a symptomatic insulinoma and reported no recurrence of hypogly-
cemic symptoms after the procedure.[121]

Recently, Choi and colleagues reported a large-scale study of EUS-guided ethanol
ablation for solid pancreatic tumors. EUS-guided ethanol ablation was performed in
72 patients with solid pancreatic tumors (47 with PNETs and 25 with SPTs). Over a

| Table 3 | |
Evolution of endoscopic local tumor therapy for pancreas and biliary neoplasm	
	Author, Year
EUS-EL for PCNs	Gan et al,[119] 2005
EUS-EL with paclitaxel injection for PCNs	Oh, et al,[120] 2008
EUS-guided ethanol ablation in an elderly patient with symptomatic insulinoma	Jurgensen et al,[121] 2006
RFA with benign pancreatic tumors (6 PCNs and 2 neuroendocrine tumors)	Pai et al,[123] 2015
EUS-guided fiducial placement for mediastinal or abdominal malignancies	Pishvavaian et al,[125] 2006
EUS-guided brachytherapy for unresectable pancreatic cancer	Sun et al,[128] 2006
Endo-biliary RFA for unresectable malignant biliary obstructions	Steel et al,[129] 2011
Photodynamic therapy through a choledochoscope for cholangiocarcinoma	McCaughan et al,[133] 1991

Abbreviations: EUS, endoscopic ultrasound; PCNs, pancreatic cystic neoplasms; RFA, radiofrequency ablation.

median follow-up of 18.4 months, 8 patients showed complete morphologic remission, 40 exhibited partial remission, 16 had stable disease, and 8 had progressive disease. Procedure-related AEs were noted in 31.9% of the cases, the majority of which were of mild-to-moderate severity.[122] Although results are promising in the short-to-medium term, long-term data on the effectiveness and safety of EUS-guided pancreatic tumor ablation are still needed.

Endoscopic Ultrasound-Guided Radiofrequency Ablation

Although radiofrequency ablation (RFA) is widely used for malignancies such as hepatocellular carcinoma, a high-frequency ablation probe designed for EUS has only recently been developed and is currently being used for the treatment of pancreatic tumors.

In 2015, Pai and colleagues first described high-frequency thermal ablation using the Habib probe in 8 patients with benign pancreatic tumors (6 PCNs and 2 PNETs).[123] The results showed complete remission in 2 patients with PCNs, whereas the remaining 4 patients experienced an average tumor size reduction of 48.4%. In the 2 patients with PNETs, a postprocedure examination revealed necrosis within the tumors.

Endoscopic Ultrasound-Guided Radiotherapy

Stereotactic body radiation therapy (SBRT) delivers high-dose radiation to the tumor area. Compared with conventional radiation therapy, SBRT has a shorter treatment duration and is more effective for unresectable pancreatic cancer.[124] The fiducial marker inserted at the margin of a pancreatic tumor acts as a fixed reference point within the tumor, aiding in overcoming target movement during precise radiation therapy. Traditionally, fiducial markers have been percutaneously inserted under CT or ultrasound guidance. However, percutaneous fiducial marker insertion carries a higher risk of vascular injury and reduces the accuracy owing to the retroperitoneal position of the pancreas. In 2006, EUS-guided fiducial placement was first described by Pishvavaian and colleagues and was successfully performed in 11 of 13 patients with mediastinal or abdominal malignancies.[125] In a relatively large-scale retrospective study involving 57 consecutive patients, 50 underwent successful EUS-guided gold fiducial placement for image-guided radiation treatment, with only one minor bleeding event.[126] EUS-guided fiducial marker placement is an essential step in preparing patients with locally advanced pancreatic cancer for SBRT.

Brachytherapy involves the insertion of a radioactive source into or near the tumor tissue to facilitate tumor treatment. The radioactive sources used in brachytherapy include iodine-125, iridium-192, or palladium-103. Iodine-125 is beneficial for rapidly growing pancreatic cancers because of its long half-life. Sun and colleagues demonstrated through animal experiments that radioactive sources could be safely inserted into the pancreas using EUS.[127] In 2006, a pilot study of EUS-guided brachytherapy involving 15 patients with unresectable pancreatic cancer, 12 maintained a stable or partial response and 30% of the patients showed clinical improvement such as pain reduction.[128] Improved outcomes are expected with the development of new radioactive sources.

Endo-Biliary Radiofrequency Ablation

Intraductal RFA for treatment of malignant biliary obstruction is performed using ERCP or percutaneous transhepatic cholangiography. In 2011, Steel and colleagues introduced endobiliary RFA treatment of 22 patients with unresectable malignant biliary obstructions.[129] Clinical studies on endobiliary RFA are mostly small-scale but have demonstrated technical safety and effectiveness.[130,131] Although current evidence on whether endobiliary RFA can prolong survival in malignant biliary obstruction is not conclusive, a meta-analysis by Sofi and colleagues demonstrated that the group treated with both endobiliary RFA and SEMS placement showed extended survival compared with the group that received SEMS placement only (285 days vs 248 days, $P < .001$).[132]

Endo-Biliary Photodynamic Treatment

Photodynamic therapy (PDT) uses a photosensitizer that undergoes a chemical reaction induced by light to generate singlet oxygen and free radicals. These agents selectively destroy the cancer cells without causing pain. In 1991, McCaughan and colleagues first reported the use of PDT for cholangiocarcinoma using choledochoscopy.[133] Endo-biliary PDT has been reported to improve quality of life, bile drainage, and survival rates in patients with unresectable bile duct cancer.[134,135]

PDT is limited to adjunctive treatment, ranging from palliative care for unresectable bile duct cancer to supplementary therapy for patients with incompletely resected tumors. Further clinical research is crucial to identify the most suitable candidates with cholangiocarcinoma to receive PDT.

SUMMARY

With the introduction of ERCP and linear EUS, interventional PB endoscopy has had an enormous impact in the management of pancreatic and biliary diseases. Continuous efforts to improve various devices and techniques have revolutionized these treatment modalities as viable alternatives to surgery. In recent years, trends toward combining endoscopic techniques with other modalities, such as laparoscopic and radiological interventions, for complex PB diseases have emerged using a multidisciplinary approach. Ongoing research and clinical experience will lead to refinements in interventional PB endoscopic techniques and subsequently improve outcomes and reduce complication rates.

CLINICS CARE POINTS

- Advancements in bile duct stone treatment, including EST with ERCP, EPLBD, ML, and various stone removal techniques such as LL and EHL under peroral cholangioscopy, have significantly improved outcomes.

- Mechanical dilation, naso-biliary drainage, and PS or SEMS placement have significantly advanced the treatment of benign and malignant biliary strictures. In MHBO, unilateral drainage may be sufficient; however, high-grade obstructions require bilateral or multiple drainage procedures, which can be technically challenging. EUS-BD, such as EUS-CDS, EUS-HGS, EUS-HDS, or EUS-RV, offers additional options for cases of unsuccessful ERCP.

- The evolution of EUS-GBD has significantly improved clinical outcomes, surpassing those of conventional methods and percutaneous cholecystostomy in terms of reintervention rates.

- EST, ENBD, and PS placement have become pivotal for managing bile leaks. FCSEMS placement offers a valuable alternative, especially for complex cases or refractory leaks.

- EUS-guided drainage has revolutionized the treatment of PP and WON by providing minimally invasive alternatives to surgery. The "step-up" approach has emerged as the preferred strategy for infected WON.

- Management of PD leaks with or without DPDS has evolved from traditional surgical interventions to less-invasive approaches such as transpapillary PD stenting with ERCP, EUS-guided interventions, radiologic interventions, or a combination.

- Use of colonoscopes, transparent caps, SBE, and DBE has improved the success rate of ERCP in patients with SAA. More recently, EUS-guided directed transgastric ERCP using LAMS placement has emerged as a promising method, eliminating the need for DBE or SBE, reducing procedure time, and significantly increasing success rates compared with traditional approaches.

DISCLOSURE

The authors have no financial disclosures.

SUPPLEMENTARY DATA

Supplementary data related to this article can be found online at https://doi.org/10.1016/j.giec.2023.12.001.

REFERENCES

1. Schuman BM. The evolution of diagnostic ERCP. Gastrointest Endosc 1990; 36(2):155–6.
2. Binmoeller KF. Optimizing interventional EUS: the echoendoscope in evolution. Gastrointest Endosc 2007;66(5):917–9.
3. McCune WS, Shorb PE, Moscovitz H. Endoscopic cannulation of the ampulla of vater: a preliminary report. Ann Surg 1968;167(5):752–6.
4. Classen M, Demling L. [Endoscopic sphincterotomy of the papilla of vater and extraction of stones from the choledochal duct (author's transl)]. Dtsch Med Wochenschr 1974;99(11):496–7. Endoskopische Sphinkterotomie der Papilla Vateri und Steinextraktion aus dem Ductus choledochus.
5. Kawai K, Akasaka Y, Murakami K, et al. Endoscopic sphincterotomy of the ampulla of Vater. Gastrointest Endosc 1974;20(4):148–51.
6. Leuschner U. Endoscopic therapy of biliary calculi. Clin Gastroenterol 1986; 15(2):333–58.
7. Sivak MV Jr. Endoscopic management of bile duct stones. Am J Surg 1989; 158(3):228–40.
8. Riemann JF, Seuberth K, Demling L. Clinical application of a new mechanical lithotripter for smashing common bile duct stones. Endoscopy 1982;14(6): 226–30.
9. Shaw MJ, Mackie RD, Moore JP, et al. Results of a multicenter trial using a mechanical lithotripter for the treatment of large bile duct stones. Am J Gastroenterol 1993;88(5):730–3.
10. Garg PK, Tandon RK, Ahuja V, et al. Predictors of unsuccessful mechanical lithotripsy and endoscopic clearance of large bile duct stones. Gastrointest Endosc 2004;59(6):601–5.
11. Koch H, Stolte M, Walz V. Endoscopic lithotripsy in the common bile duct. Endoscopy 1977;9(2):95–8.
12. Lux G, Ell C, Hochberger J, et al. The first successful endoscopic retrograde laser lithotripsy of common bile duct stones in man using a pulsed neodymium-YAG laser. Endoscopy 1986;18(4):144–5.
13. Chen YK, Parsi MA, Binmoeller KF, et al. Single-operator cholangioscopy in patients requiring evaluation of bile duct disease or therapy of biliary stones (with videos). Gastrointest Endosc 2011;74(4):805–14.

14. Korrapati P, Ciolino J, Wani S, et al. The efficacy of peroral cholangioscopy for difficult bile duct stones and indeterminate strictures: a systematic review and meta-analysis. Endosc Int Open 2016;4(3):E263–75.

15. Ersoz G, Tekesin O, Ozutemiz AO, et al. Biliary sphincterotomy plus dilation with a large balloon for bile duct stones that are difficult to extract. Gastrointest Endosc 2003;57(2):156–9.

16. Kim TH, Oh HJ, Lee JY, et al. Can a small endoscopic sphincterotomy plus a large-balloon dilation reduce the use of mechanical lithotripsy in patients with large bile duct stones? Surg Endosc 2011;25(10):3330–7.

17. Attasaranya S, Cheon YK, Vittal H, et al. Large-diameter biliary orifice balloon dilation to aid in endoscopic bile duct stone removal: a multicenter series. Gastrointest Endosc 2008;67(7):1046–52.

18. Heo JH, Kang DH, Jung HJ, et al. Endoscopic sphincterotomy plus large-balloon dilation versus endoscopic sphincterotomy for removal of bile-duct stones. Gastrointest Endosc 2007;66(4):720–6, quiz 768, 771.

19. Maydeo A, Bhandari S. Balloon sphincteroplasty for removing difficult bile duct stones. Endoscopy 2007;39(11):958–61.

20. Burhenne HJ, Morris DC. Biliary stricture dilatation: use of the Gruntzig balloon catheter. J Can Assoc Radiol 1980;31(3):196–7.

21. Judah JR, Draganov PV. Endoscopic therapy of benign biliary strictures. World J Gastroenterol 2007;13(26):3531–9.

22. Nagai N, Toli F, Oi I, et al. Continuous endoscopic pancreatocholedochal catheterization. Gastrointest Endosc 1976;23(2):78–81.

23. Wurbs D, Phillip J, Classen M. Experiences with the long standing nasobiliary tube in biliary diseases. Endoscopy 1980;12(5):219–23.

24. Soehendra N, Reynders-Frederix V. [Palliative biliary duct drainage. A new method for endoscopic introduction of a new drain]. Dtsch Med Wochenschr 1979;104(6):206–7. Palliative Gallengangdrainage. Eine neue Methode zur endoskopischen Einfuhrung eines inneren Drains.

25. Huibregtse K, Cheng J, Coene PP, et al. Endoscopic placement of expandable metal stents for biliary strictures–a preliminary report on experience with 33 patients. Endoscopy 1989;21(6):280–2.

26. Takasaki M, Morita S, Horimi T, et al. [Endoscopic placement of self-expandable metallic stents (Wallstent) for malignant biliary stenosis, with special reference to preventive endoscopic nasal bile drainage against acute obstruction after stenting]. Nihon Shokakibyo Gakkai Zasshi 1995;92(9):1275–84.

27. Zhang X, Wang X, Wang L, et al. Effect of covered self-expanding metal stents compared with multiple plastic stents on benign biliary stricture: A meta-analysis. *Medicine (Baltimore).* Sep 2018;97(36):e12039.

28. Tringali A, Barbaro F, Pizzicannella M, et al. Endoscopic management with multiple plastic stents of anastomotic biliary stricture following liver transplantation: long-term results. Endoscopy 2016;48(6):546–51.

29. Haapamaki C, Kylanpaa L, Udd M, et al. Randomized multicenter study of multiple plastic stents vs. covered self-expandable metallic stent in the treatment of biliary stricture in chronic pancreatitis. Endoscopy 2015;47(7):605–10.

30. Sbeit W, Khoury T, Goldin E, et al. Three-months duration of fully-covered metal stent for refractory dominant extra-hepatic biliary stricture among primary sclerosing cholangitis patients: efficacy and safety. Surg Endosc 2022;36(4):2412–7.

31. Jang SI, Chung TR, Cho JH, et al. Short fully covered self-expandable metal stent for treatment of proximal anastomotic benign biliary stricture after living-donor liver transplantation. Dig Endosc 2021;33(5):840–8.

32. Poley JW, Ponchon T, Puespoek A, et al. Fully covered self-expanding metal stents for benign biliary stricture after orthotopic liver transplant: 5-year outcomes. Gastrointest Endosc 2020;92(6):1216–24.

33. Kao D, Zepeda-Gomez S, Tandon P, et al. Managing the post-liver transplantation anastomotic biliary stricture: multiple plastic versus metal stents: a systematic review. Gastrointest Endosc 2013;77(5):679–91.

34. Landi F, de'Angelis N, Sepulveda A, et al. Endoscopic treatment of anastomotic biliary stricture after adult deceased donor liver transplantation with multiple plastic stents versus self-expandable metal stents: a systematic review and meta-analysis. Transpl Int 2018;31(2):131–51.

35. Elmunzer BJ, Maranki JL, Gomez V, et al. ACG Clinical Guideline: Diagnosis and Management of Biliary Strictures. Am J Gastroenterol 2023;118(3):405–26.

36. Almadi MA, Barkun A, Martel M. Plastic vs. Self-Expandable Metal Stents for Palliation in Malignant Biliary Obstruction: A Series of Meta-Analyses. Am J Gastroenterol 2017;112(2):260–73.

37. Almadi MA, Barkun AN, Martel M. No benefit of covered vs uncovered self-expandable metal stents in patients with malignant distal biliary obstruction: a meta-analysis. Clin Gastroenterol Hepatol 2013;11(1):27–37 e1.

38. Li J, Li T, Sun P, et al. Covered versus Uncovered Self-Expandable Metal Stents for Managing Malignant Distal Biliary Obstruction: A Meta-Analysis. PLoS One 2016;11(2):e0149066.

39. Tringali A, Hassan C, Rota M, et al. Covered vs. uncovered self-expandable metal stents for malignant distal biliary strictures: a systematic review and meta-analysis. Endoscopy 2018;50(6):631–41.

40. Chang WH, Kortan P, Haber GB. Outcome in patients with bifurcation tumors who undergo unilateral versus bilateral hepatic duct drainage. Gastrointest Endosc 1998;47(5):354–62.

41. Lee TH, Kim TH, Moon JH, et al. Bilateral versus unilateral placement of metal stents for inoperable high-grade malignant hilar biliary strictures: a multicenter, prospective, randomized study (with video). Gastrointest Endosc 2017;86(5):817–27.

42. Giovannini M, Moutardier V, Pesenti C, et al. Endoscopic ultrasound-guided bilioduodenal anastomosis: a new technique for biliary drainage. Endoscopy 2001;33(10):898–900.

43. Burmester E, Niehaus J, Leineweber T, et al. EUS-cholangio-drainage of the bile duct: report of 4 cases. Gastrointest Endosc 2003;57(2):246–51.

44. Mallery S, Matlock J, Freeman ML. EUS-guided rendezvous drainage of obstructed biliary and pancreatic ducts: Report of 6 cases. Gastrointest Endosc 2004;59(1):100–7.

45. Giovannini M, Dotti M, Bories E, et al. Hepaticogastrostomy by echo-endoscopy as a palliative treatment in a patient with metastatic biliary obstruction. Endoscopy 2003;35(12):1076–8.

46. Park SJ, Choi JH, Park DH, et al. Expanding indication: EUS-guided hepaticoduodenostomy for isolated right intrahepatic duct obstruction (with video). Gastrointest Endosc 2013;78(2):374–80.

47. Klair JS, Zafar Y, Ashat M, et al. Effectiveness and Safety of EUS Rendezvous After Failed Biliary Cannulation With ERCP: A Systematic Review and Proportion Meta-analysis. J Clin Gastroenterol 2023;57(2):211–7.

48. Foerster EC, Auth J, Runge U, et al. ERCG: endoscopic retrograde catheterization of the gallbladder. Endoscopy 1988;20(1):30–2.
49. Ponchon T, Baroud J, Mestas JL, et al. Gallbladder lithotripsy: retrograde dissolution of fragments. Gastrointest Endosc 1988;34(6):468–9.
50. Feretis CB, Manouras AJ, Apostolidis NS, et al. Endoscopic transpapillary drainage of gallbladder empyema. Gastrointest Endosc Sep-Oct 1990;36(5):523–5.
51. Itoi T, Coelho-Prabhu N, Baron TH. Endoscopic gallbladder drainage for management of acute cholecystitis. Gastrointest Endosc 2010;71(6):1038–45.
52. Baron TH, Topazian MD. Endoscopic transduodenal drainage of the gallbladder: implications for endoluminal treatment of gallbladder disease. Gastrointest Endosc 2007;65(4):735–7.
53. Jang JW, Lee SS, Park DH, et al. Feasibility and safety of EUS-guided transgastric/transduodenal gallbladder drainage with single-step placement of a modified covered self-expandable metal stent in patients unsuitable for cholecystectomy. Gastrointest Endosc 2011;74(1):176–81.
54. Itoi T, Binmoeller KF, Shah J, et al. Clinical evaluation of a novel lumen-apposing metal stent for endosonography-guided pancreatic pseudocyst and gallbladder drainage (with videos). Gastrointest Endosc 2012;75(4):870–6.
55. McCarty TR, Hathorn KE, Bazarbashi AN, et al. Endoscopic gallbladder drainage for symptomatic gallbladder disease: a cumulative systematic review meta-analysis. Surg Endosc 2021;35(9):4964–85.
56. Browder IW, Dowling JB, Koontz KK, et al. Early management of operative injuries of the extrahepatic biliary tract. Ann Surg 1987;205(6):649–58.
57. Kune GA. Bile duct injury during cholecystectomy: causes, prevention and surgical repair in 1979. Aust N Z J Surg 1979;49(1):35–40.
58. Taylor JD, Carr-Locke DL, Fossard DP. Bile peritonitis and hemobilia after percutaneous liver biopsy: endoscopic retrograde cholangiopancreatography demonstration of bile leak. Am J Gastroenterol 1987;82(3):262–4.
59. Smith AC, Schapiro RH, Kelsey PB, et al. Successful treatment of nonhealing biliary-cutaneous fistulas with biliary stents. Gastroenterology 1986;90(3):764–9.
60. O'Rahilly S, Duignan JP, Lennon JR, et al. Successful treatment of a postoperative external biliary fistula by endoscopic papillotomy. Endoscopy 1983;15(2):68–9.
61. Kozarek RA, Ball TJ, Patterson DJ, et al. Endoscopic treatment of biliary injury in the era of laparoscopic cholecystectomy. Gastrointest Endosc 1994;40(1):10–6.
62. Baron TH, Poterucha JJ. Insertion and removal of covered expandable metal stents for closure of complex biliary leaks. Clin Gastroenterol Hepatol 2006;4(3):381–6.
63. Canena J, Liberato M, Meireles L, et al. A non-randomized study in consecutive patients with postcholecystectomy refractory biliary leaks who were managed endoscopically with the use of multiple plastic stents or fully covered self-expandable metal stents (with videos). Gastrointest Endosc 2015;82(1):70–8.
64. Banks PA, Bollen TL, Dervenis C, et al. Classification of acute pancreatitis–2012: revision of the Atlanta classification and definitions by international consensus. Gut 2013;62(1):102–11.
65. Mousseau LP, Kling S. Pancreatic pseudocyst. Can Med Assoc J 1948;59(6):550–4.
66. MacErlean DP, Bryan PJ, Murphy JJ. Pancreatic pseudocyst: management by ultrasonically guided aspiration. Gastrointest Radiol 1980;5(3):255–7.

67. Bernardino ME, Amerson JR. Percutaneous gastrocystostomy: a new approach to pancreatic pseudocyst drainage. AJR Am J Roentgenol 1984;143(5):1096–7.
68. Ho CS, Taylor B. Percutaneous transgastric drainage for pancreatic pseudocyst. AJR Am J Roentgenol 1984;143(3):623–5.
69. Rogers BH, Cicurel NJ, Seed RW. Transgastric needle aspiration of pancreatic pseudocyst through an endoscope. Gastrointest Endosc 1975;21(3):133–4.
70. Kozarek RA, Brayko CM, Harlan J, et al. Endoscopic drainage of pancreatic pseudocysts. Gastrointest Endosc 1985;31(5):322–7.
71. Grimm H, Binmoeller KF, Soehendra N. Endosonography-guided drainage of a pancreatic pseudocyst. Gastrointest Endosc 1992;38(2):170–1.
72. Wiersema MJ. Endosonography-guided cystoduodenostomy with a therapeutic ultrasound endoscope. Gastrointest Endosc 1996;44(5):614–7.
73. Kahaleh M, Shami VM, Conaway MR, et al. Endoscopic ultrasound drainage of pancreatic pseudocyst: a prospective comparison with conventional endoscopic drainage. Endoscopy 2006;38(4):355–9.
74. Varadarajulu S, Christein JD, Tamhane A, et al. Prospective randomized trial comparing EUS and EGD for transmural drainage of pancreatic pseudocysts (with videos). Gastrointest Endosc 2008;68(6):1102–11.
75. Baron TH, Thaggard WG, Morgan DE, et al. Endoscopic therapy for organized pancreatic necrosis. Gastroenterology 1996;111(3):755–64.
76. Seifert H, Wehrmann T, Schmitt T, et al. Retroperitoneal endoscopic debridement for infected peripancreatic necrosis. Lancet 2000;356(9230):653–5.
77. Seifert H, Biermer M, Schmitt W, et al. Transluminal endoscopic necrosectomy after acute pancreatitis: a multicentre study with long-term follow-up (the GEPARD Study). Gut 2009;58(9):1260–6.
78. Gardner TB, Chahal P, Papachristou GI, et al. A comparison of direct endoscopic necrosectomy with transmural endoscopic drainage for the treatment of walled-off pancreatic necrosis. Gastrointest Endosc 2009;69(6):1085–94.
79. Yasuda I, Nakashima M, Iwai T, et al. Japanese multicenter experience of endoscopic necrosectomy for infected walled-off pancreatic necrosis: The JENIPaN study. Endoscopy 2013;45(8):627–34.
80. van Santvoort HC, Besselink MG, Bakker OJ, et al. A step-up approach or open necrosectomy for necrotizing pancreatitis. N Engl J Med 2010;362(16):1491–502.
81. Bakker OJ, van Santvoort HC, van Brunschot S, et al. Endoscopic transgastric vs surgical necrosectomy for infected necrotizing pancreatitis: a randomized trial. JAMA 2012;307(10):1053–61.
82. Kozarek RA, Ball TJ, Patterson DJ, et al. Endoscopic transpapillary therapy for disrupted pancreatic duct and peripancreatic fluid collections. Gastroenterology 1991;100(5 Pt 1):1362–70.
83. Saeed ZA, Ramirez FC, Hepps KS. Endoscopic stent placement for internal and external pancreatic fistulas. Gastroenterology 1993;105(4):1213–7.
84. Telford JJ, Farrell JJ, Saltzman JR, et al. Pancreatic stent placement for duct disruption. Gastrointest Endosc 2002;56(1):18–24.
85. Deviere J, Bueso H, Baize M, et al. Complete disruption of the main pancreatic duct: endoscopic management. Gastrointest Endosc 1995;42(5):445–51.
86. Varadarajulu S, Wilcox CM. Endoscopic placement of permanent indwelling transmural stents in disconnected pancreatic duct syndrome: does benefit outweigh the risks? Gastrointest Endosc 2011;74(6):1408–12.

87. Arvanitakis M, Delhaye M, Bali MA, et al. Pancreatic-fluid collections: a random-ized controlled trial regarding stent removal after endoscopic transmural drainage. Gastrointest Endosc 2007;65(4):609–19.

88. Lawrence C, Howell DA, Stefan AM, et al. Disconnected pancreatic tail syn-drome: potential for endoscopic therapy and results of long-term follow-up. Gastrointest Endosc 2008;67(4):673–9.

89. Baron TH, Harewood GC, Morgan DE, et al. Outcome differences after endo-scopic drainage of pancreatic necrosis, acute pancreatic pseudocysts, and chronic pancreatic pseudocysts. Gastrointest Endosc 2002;56(1):7–17.

90. Haggard WD, Kirtley JA. Pancreatic Calculi: A Review of Sixty-Five Operative and One Hundred Thirty-Nine Non-Operative Cases. Ann Surg 1939;109(5): 809–26.

91. Inui K, Nakae Y, Nakamura J, et al. A case of non-calcified pancreatolithiasis which was removed by endoscopic sphincterotomy of the pancreatic duct. Gas-troenterol Endosc 1983;25(8):1246–53.

92. Fuji T, Amano H, Harima K, et al. Pancreatic sphincterotomy and pancreatic en-doprosthesis. Endoscopy 1985;17(2):69–72.

93. Sauerbruch T, Holl J, Sackmann M, et al. Disintegration of a pancreatic duct stone with extracorporeal shock waves in a patient with chronic pancreatitis. Endoscopy 1987;19(5):207–8.

94. van der Hul R, Plaisier P, Jeekel J, et al. Extracorporeal shock-wave lithotripsy of pancreatic duct stones: immediate and long-term results. Endoscopy 1994; 26(7):573–8.

95. Adamek HE, Jakobs R, Buttmann A, et al. Long term follow up of patients with chronic pancreatitis and pancreatic stones treated with extracorporeal shock wave lithotripsy. Gut 1999;45(3):402–5.

96. Inui K, Tazuma S, Yamaguchi T, et al. Treatment of pancreatic stones with extra-corporeal shock wave lithotripsy: results of a multicenter survey. Pancreas 2005; 30(1):26–30.

97. Hu LH, Ye B, Yang YG, et al. Extracorporeal Shock Wave Lithotripsy for Chinese Patients With Pancreatic Stones: A Prospective Study of 214 Cases. Pancreas 2016;45(2):298–305.

98. Choi KS, Kim MH. Extracorporeal shock wave lithotripsy for the treatment of pancreatic duct stones. J Hepatobiliary Pancreat Surg 2006;13(2):86–93.

99. Kozarek RA, Brandabur JJ, Ball TJ, et al. Clinical outcomes in patients who un-dergo extracorporeal shock wave lithotripsy for chronic calcific pancreatitis. Gastrointest Endosc 2002;56(4):496–500.

100. Howell DA, Dy RM, Hanson BL, et al. Endoscopic treatment of pancreatic duct stones using a 10F pancreatoscope and electrohydraulic lithotripsy. Gastroint-est Endosc 1999;50(6):829–33.

101. Costamagna G, Bulajic M, Tringali A, et al. Multiple stenting of refractory pancre-atic duct strictures in severe chronic pancreatitis: long-term results. Endoscopy 2006;38(3):254–9.

102. Dite P, Ruzicka M, Zboril V, et al. A prospective, randomized trial comparing endoscopic and surgical therapy for chronic pancreatitis. Endoscopy 2003; 35(7):553–8.

103. Eisendrath P, Deviere J. Expandable metal stents for benign pancreatic duct obstruction. Gastrointest Endosc Clin N Am 1999;9(3):547–54.

104. Park DH, Kim MH, Moon SH, et al. Feasibility and safety of placement of a newly designed, fully covered self-expandable metal stent for refractory benign

pancreatic ductal strictures: a pilot study (with video). Gastrointest Endosc 2008;68(6):1182–9.

105. Oh D, Lee JH, Song TJ, et al. Long-term outcomes of 6-mm diameter fully covered self-expandable metal stents in benign refractory pancreatic ductal stricture. Dig Endosc 2018;30(4):508–15.

106. Shami VM, Kahaleh M. Endoscopic ultrasonography (EUS)-guided access and therapy of pancreatico-biliary disorders: EUS-guided cholangio and pancreatic drainage. Gastrointest Endosc Clin N Am 2007;17(3):581–93, vii-viii.

107. Eisenberg E, Carr DB, Chalmers TC. Neurolytic celiac plexus block for treatment of cancer pain: a meta-analysis. Anesth Analg 1995;80(2):290–5.

108. Wiersema MJ, Wiersema LM. Endosonography-guided celiac plexus neurolysis. Gastrointest Endosc 1996;44(6):656–62.

109. Gunaratnam NT, Sarma AV, Norton ID, et al. A prospective study of EUS-guided celiac plexus neurolysis for pancreatic cancer pain. Gastrointest Endosc 2001; 54(3):316–24.

110. Katon RM, Bilbao MK, Parent JA, et al. Endoscopic retrograde cholangiopan-creatography in patients with gastrectomy and gastrojejunostomy (Billroth II), A case for the forward look. Gastrointest Endosc 1975;21(4):164–5.

111. Gostout CJ, Bender CE. Cholangiopancreatography, sphincterotomy, and common duct stone removal via Roux-en-Y limb enteroscopy. Gastroenterology 1988;95(1):156–63.

112. Yamamoto H, Sekine Y, Sato Y, et al. Total enteroscopy with a nonsurgical steer-able double-balloon method. Gastrointest Endosc 2001;53(2):216–20.

113. Monkemuller K, Fry LC, Bellutti M, et al. ERCP using single-balloon instead of double-balloon enteroscopy in patients with Roux-en-Y anastomosis. Endos-copy 2008;40(Suppl 2):E19–20.

114. Saleem A, Baron TH, Gostout CJ, et al. Endoscopic retrograde cholangiopan-creatography using a single-balloon enteroscope in patients with altered Roux-en-Y anatomy. Endoscopy 2010;42(8):656–60.

115. Baron TH, Vickers SM. Surgical gastrostomy placement as access for diag-nostic and therapeutic ERCP. Gastrointest Endosc 1998;48(6):640–1.

116. Peters M, Papasavas PK, Caushaj PF, et al. Laparoscopic transgastric endo-scopic retrograde cholangiopancreatography for benign common bile duct stricture after Roux-en-Y gastric bypass. Surg Endosc 2002;16(7):1106.

117. Vallabh H, Poushanchi B, Hsueh W, et al. EUS-directed transgastric ERCP (EDGE) with use of a 20-mm x 10-mm lumen-apposing metal stent in a patient with Roux-en-Y gastric bypass. VideoGIE 2018;3(9):262–3.

118. Bukhari M, Kowalski T, Nieto J, et al. An international, multicenter, comparative trial of EUS-guided gastrogastrostomy-assisted ERCP versus enteroscopy-assisted ERCP in patients with Roux-en-Y gastric bypass anatomy. Gastrointest Endosc 2018;88(3):486–94.

119. Gan SI, Thompson CC, Lauwers GY, et al. Ethanol lavage of pancreatic cystic lesions: initial pilot study. Gastrointest Endosc 2005;61(6):746–52.

120. Oh HC, Seo DW, Lee TY, et al. New treatment for cystic tumors of the pancreas: EUS-guided ethanol lavage with paclitaxel injection. Gastrointest Endosc 2008; 67(4):636–42.

121. Jurgensen C, Schuppan D, Neser F, et al. EUS-guided alcohol ablation of an in-sulinoma. Gastrointest Endosc 2006;63(7):1059–62.

122. Choi JH, Paik WH, Lee SH, et al. Efficacy and predictive factors of endoscopic ultrasound-guided ethanol ablation in benign solid pancreatic tumors. Surg En-dosc 2023;37(8):5960–8.

123. Pai M, Habib N, Senturk H, et al. Endoscopic ultrasound guided radiofrequency ablation, for pancreatic cystic neoplasms and neuroendocrine tumors. World J Gastrointest Surg 2015;7(4):52–9.
124. Chang DT, Schellenberg D, Shen J, et al. Stereotactic radiotherapy for unresectable adenocarcinoma of the pancreas. Cancer 2009;115(3):665–72.
125. Pishvaian AC, Collins B, Gagnon G, et al. EUS-guided fiducial placement for CyberKnife radiotherapy of mediastinal and abdominal malignancies. Gastrointest Endosc 2006;64(3):412–7.
126. Park WG, Yan BM, Schellenberg D, et al. EUS-guided gold fiducial insertion for image-guided radiation therapy of pancreatic cancer: 50 successful cases without fluoroscopy. Gastrointest Endosc 2010;71(3):513–8.
127. Sun S, Qingjie L, Qiyong G, et al. EUS-guided interstitial brachytherapy of the pancreas: a feasibility study. Gastrointest Endosc 2005;62(5):775–9.
128. Sun S, Xu H, Xin J, et al. Endoscopic ultrasound-guided interstitial brachytherapy of unresectable pancreatic cancer: results of a pilot trial. Endoscopy 2006;38(4):399–403.
129. Steel AW, Postgate AJ, Khorsandi S, et al. Endoscopically applied radiofrequency ablation appears to be safe in the treatment of malignant biliary obstruction. Gastrointest Endosc 2011;73(1):149–53.
130. Alis H, Sengoz C, Gonenc M, et al. Endobiliary radiofrequency ablation for malignant biliary obstruction. Hepatobiliary Pancreat Dis Int 2013;12(4):423–7.
131. Inoue T, Ibusuki M, Kitano R, et al. Endobiliary radiofrequency ablation combined with bilateral metal stent placement for malignant hilar biliary obstruction. Endoscopy 2020;52(7):595–9.
132. Sofi AA, Khan MA, Das A, et al. Radiofrequency ablation combined with biliary stent placement versus stent placement alone for malignant biliary strictures: a systematic review and meta-analysis. Gastrointest Endosc 2018;87(4): 944–951 e1.
133. McCaughan JS Jr, Mertens BF, Cho C, et al. Photodynamic therapy to treat tumors of the extrahepatic biliary ducts. A case report. Arch Surg 1991;126(1): 111–3.
134. Ortner MA, Liebetruth J, Schreiber S, et al. Photodynamic therapy of nonresectable cholangiocarcinoma. Gastroenterology 1998;114(3):536–42.
135. Ortner M. Photodynamic therapy for cholangiocarcinoma. J Hepatobiliary Pancreat Surg 2001;8(2):137–9.

Endoscopic Retrograde Cholangiopancreatography for the Management of Pancreatic Duct Leaks and Fistulas

Hadie Razjouyan, MD, Jennifer L. Maranki, MD, MSc*

KEYWORDS

- Pancreatitis • Pancreatic duct leak • Pancreatic fistula • ERCP • Pancreatic stent

KEY POINTS

- Pancreatic duct leaks are a common complication of acute and chronic pancreatitis, trauma to the pancreas, and pancreatic surgery.
- Diagnosis of PD leaks and fistulas is often made with contrast-enhanced pancreatic protocol computed tomography or magnetic resonance imaging with MRCP.
- Endoscopic retrograde pancreatography with pancreatic duct stenting in appropriately selected patients is often an effective treatment, helps to avoid surgery, and is considered first-line therapy in cases that fail conservative management.

INTRODUCTION

Pancreatic duct leaks may arise in the setting of acute or chronic pancreatitis, as a result of pancreatic trauma, or surgical manipulation. In acute pancreatitis, the inflammatory process causes damage to the pancreatic ductal epithelium resulting in a leak, which may manifest as an acute fluid collection or pseudocyst. In chronic pancreatitis, typically an obstructing pancreatic duct stone and/or ductal stenosis results in elevated pressures in the upstream duct, resulting in trauma to the duct and the development of a leak or fistula.

Pancreatic leaks and fistulas are typically classified as either external or internal.[1] External leaks are pancreaticocutaneous fistulas and usually occur as a result of pancreatic surgery or trauma and following percutaneous drainage of pancreatic fluid collections. Internal leaks present in a variety of ways, including pancreatic ascites, pseudocysts, or pleural effusions. Both types of fistulas are associated with significant morbidity.

Division of Gastroenterology and Hepatology, Penn State College of Medicine, Penn State Health, 500 University Drive, HU850, Hershey, PA 17033, USA
* Corresponding author.
E-mail address: jmaranki@pennstatehealth.psu.edu

Gastrointest Endoscopy Clin N Am 34 (2024) 405–416
https://doi.org/10.1016/j.giec.2024.02.001
1052-5157/24/© 2024 Elsevier Inc. All rights reserved.

BACKGROUND

Acute fluid collections occur in approximately 40% of patients with acute pancreatitis. However, most of these resolve without intervention, and only a small proportion develop a fistula requiring intervention.[2,3] Any cause of pancreatitis may contribute to the development of a leak or fistula. Whether a fistula develops is generally dependent on the type and severity of the injury, and collections with pancreatic necrosis are commonly associated with a pancreatic duct leak.[4]

NATURE OF PROBLEM

Pancreatic leakage and the subsequent development of fistulas result from compromised structural integrity of the main pancreatic duct or parenchymal injury through the disruption of side branches. Such significant pancreatic injuries may manifest as partial or complete disruptions. Over time, these leaks may evolve and develop into a confined collection or create connections with new epithelialized organs, culminating in the formation of fistulas. These fistulas may vary in terms of their location, being either internal or external, and in complexity, presenting as simple (involving a single tract) or complex (involving multiple tracts).[5] The most common causes of injuries that initiate the clinical cascade mentioned above are usually benign. These injuries may result from acute or chronic pancreatitis, postsurgical complications, or trauma.[6] However, it has been reported in precancerous and cancerous conditions such as secondary to main duct intraductal papillary mucinous neoplasm (IPMN) or pancreatic cancer. Among benign causes of pancreatic enzyme leaks, disruption in the setting of necrotizing pancreatitis or recurrent acute pancreatitis is the most frequent culprits, followed by iatrogenic postoperative, 10% to 28%,[7] and trauma, less than 2% of blunt trauma cases,[8–10] **Box 1**.

When a pancreatic leak occurs, it typically tracks laterally (toward the spleen), medially (toward the duodenum or bile duct), into the lesser sac, and superiorly into the mediastinum through the diaphragmatic hiatus around the aorta and esophagus, causing a pleural or pericardial effusion.[9,11] It may also extend into the abdominal cavity and cause pancreatic ascites. The outcome largely depends on the severity of the initial insult, with most cases being self-limited or evolving into a pseudocyst or walled-off necrosis. Chronic pressure from the fluid collection and/or secondary infection can lead to decompression of the collection into surrounding organs, resulting in a spontaneous internal fistula. These internal fistulas are defined as abnormal communication between 2 epithelial surfaces.[5,12] In addition to internal fistulas, leaks can also track to the skin and cause an external (pancreato-cutaneous) fistula. These are typically associated with prior surgical or percutaneous drainage of pancreatic fluid collections.[9]

Box 1
Causes of pancreatic duct leak

Benign (most common)
- Necrotizing pancreatitis or recurrent acute pancreatitis
- Iatrogenic postoperative
- Trauma

Premalignant or malignant
- Intraductal Papillary Mucinous Neoplasm (IPMN)
- Pancreatic cancer

Fistulas are most commonly internal and could be pancreato-enteral, pancreato-pleural, pancreatic bronchial, or pancreato-peritoneal presenting as ascites. Among pancreato-enteral fistula, the most common locations are the transverse colon and duodenum,[13,14] **Box 2, Fig. 1A, B.**

EPIDEMIOLOGY

In a prospective study conducted by Uomo and colleagues, endoscopic retrograde cholangiopancreatography (ERCP) was performed within 1 week of admission in patients with biliary pancreatitis. They found a 30.5% incidence of main pancreatic duct leaks.[15] Another retrospective study, which used ERCP and/or magnetic resonance cholangiopancreatography (MRCP), reported a 38% incidence of main pancreatic duct disruption in patients with acute necrotizing pancreatitis.[16] While this is a relatively high percentage, only a small proportion of these patients will go on to develop true fistulas.[10] Among these fistulas, gastrointestinal fistulas are a common occurrence, with the transverse colon and duodenum being the most frequently affected sites.[13,14] Pleural effusion, which may be either transudative or exudative and is mostly observed on the left side, occurs in 4% to 6% of patients. However, true pancreatico-pleural fistulas are relatively rare, appearing in only 0.4% of cases, typically in patients with chronic pancreatitis experiencing exacerbations.[17,18] Risk factors for internal pancreatic fistulas include male gender, alcohol abuse, the severity of acute pancreatitis, and infected pancreatic narcosis.[12]

CLINICAL MANIFESTATIONS

The clinical manifestation of a pancreatic duct (PD) leak is primarily determined by several factors, including the location within the gland, the size of the disruption, its destination, the body's ability to contain the leak's output, and whether this confined collection is exerting pressure on surrounding organs or has become infected. Patient symptoms and signs can range from being clinically insignificant to severe complications resulting from external compression such as pain, reduced oral intake, jaundice, systemic inflammatory response syndrome, or sepsis.[10,19] As the disease progresses, and if it evolves into a fistula, the affected secondary organ becomes a source of clinical presentation. The most serious complications from pancreatic fistulas are sepsis and hemorrhage. Approximately 60% of pancreatico-enteric fistula present with GI bleeding.[12,14,20] In patients with pancreatic-pleural fistulae, the most common presentation includes dyspnea (65%–76%), followed by symptoms such as cough, chest pain, abdominal pain, and fever.[12,21]

Box 2
Case study 1

A 51-year-old gentleman presented with gallstone pancreatitis complicated by a large walled-off pancreatic necrosis (WOPN) at the head of the pancreas. This necrosis exerted compression effects on the bile duct and the antral segment of the stomach, leading to both jaundice and symptoms of gastric outlet obstruction. The patient underwent endoscopic cystgastrostomy, resulting in the resolution of jaundice and relief from gastric outlet obstruction symptoms. Subsequently, two sessions of transmural necrosectomies were performed through the cystgastrostomy. During the second necrosectomy, the patient was noted to have an internal fistula from the cyst cavity into the first portion of the duodenum (see **Fig. 1**).

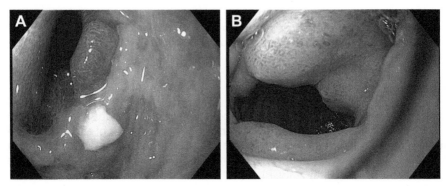

Fig. 1. Endoscopic pictures of complicated walled-off pancreatic necrosis: (*A*) Opening of the internal fistula from the cavity into the duodenal bulb. (*B*) View of the internal fistula orifice from the duodenum.

PARACLINICAL

Although historically, endoscopic retrograde pancreatography (ERP) has been the preferred method for detecting a leak and fistula, advancements in noninvasive modalities and the development of new techniques have largely replaced the diagnostic role of ERP. A pancreatic protocol contrast-enhanced CT scan is typically the initial diagnostic test of choice for patients with smoldering or severe pancreatitis who may have a pancreatic duct leak.[22] The presence of a fluid collection on a CT scan is suggestive of a leak.[10] Signs such as an edematous and indistinct gut wall or the presence of air in the pancreatic bed can raise the suspicion of a pancreatico-enteric fistula[14,23,24] in addition to an infected collection. However, due to decompression of the pancreatic duct in the case of a large fluid collection and its mass effect, along with peri-pancreatic stranding, the precise detection of duct leaks by CT scan may be suboptimal,[25] with a sensitivity of approximately 63%.[26] Magnetic resonance imaging with magnetic resonance cholangiopancreatography (MRCP) allows a reliable noninvasive pancreatography to assess PD leaks and fistulas.[27] The addition of secretin to MRCP can provide dynamic imaging to better assess the leak or fistula and guide intervention or evaluate its adequacy.[28] This modality boasts a sensitivity of up to 83%[28] and may be particularly useful in detecting areas beyond the leak or stricture, which can be challenging to assess during ERP. It is worth noting that ERP's sensitivity in diagnosing leaks ranges from 75% to 100%,[8,25] making it the gold standard for diagnosing pancreatic leaks, especially for assessing small leaks or those located in the tail of the pancreas.[29]

In cases whereby a pancreaticopleural fistula (PPF) or pancreatic ascites is suspected, fluid aspiration for analysis can provide valuable diagnostic insights. The presence of elevated amylase (>1000 U/L) and high protein levels (>3.0 g/dL) in pleural fluid is pathognomonic for PPF. However, it is crucial to rule out other potential causes of elevated amylase and protein such as tuberculosis and malignancies.[12,17,18,30] Notably, low pleural fluid protein levels do not necessarily rule out PPF, especially in malnourished patients. In peritoneal analysis, amylase levels exceeding 4000 U/L may suggest pancreatico-peritoneal ascites.

According to the International Study Group for Pancreatic Fistula (ISGPF), pancreatic leaks following pancreatic resection are classified from A to C. Grade A represents a biochemical leak, defined as any measurable drain output occurring on or after postoperative day 3, with an amylase level exceeding three times the upper limit of normal for each specific institution. Grade B is assigned when the drain has been in place for at least 3 weeks with ongoing high output and/or elevated amylase levels. Grade C is when a patient develops organ failure or requires reoperation.[31]

MANAGEMENT

This review primarily focuses on the implications of endoscopic retrograde pancreatography (ERP) in the treatment of pancreatic duct leaks and fistula (**Figs. 2** and **3**). Given the complexity of these cases and the variations in approaches, the management of patients with PD leaks or fistula are ideally discussed in multidisciplinary conferences. The appropriate treatment must be individualized and is likely to include endoscopic, percutaneous, and/or surgical techniques. These conferences often involve pancreaticobiliary surgeons, diagnostic and interventional radiologists, and interventional endoscopists who actively engage in the management of these cases. For information regarding disconnected duct syndrome, please refer to the dedicated article.

In the early phase of pancreatic leak, meaning the first 2 to 4 weeks when the fluid collection is amorphous without an organized wall, the primary approach is conservative management. These measures typically initially involve bowel rest, followed by supplemental feeding, either via nasojejunal tube feeds or total parenteral nutrition, and potentially the use of octreotide.

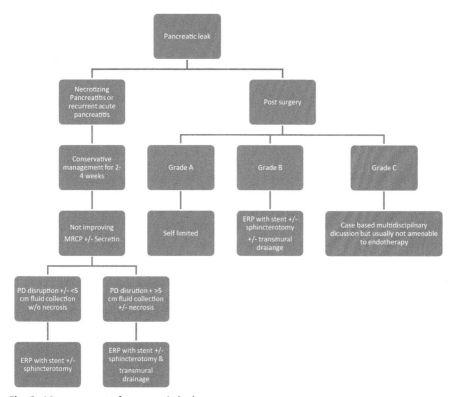

Fig. 2. Management of pancreatic leak.

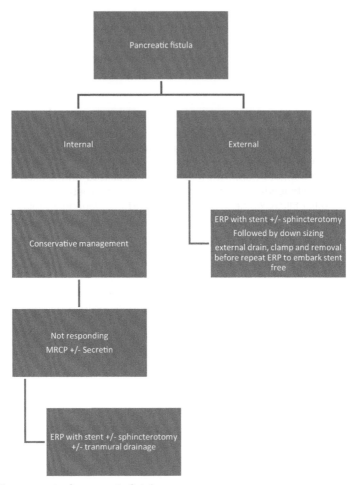

Fig. 3. Management of pancreatic fistula.

After the first few weeks, if there is a lack of clinical improvement, ERP provides the ability to perform a pancreatic sphincterotomy as well as place a pancreatic duct stent, thereby facilitating the closure of the leak. Pancreatic duct stent placement was reported by Kozarek and colleagues 30 years ago when they reported their case series of 4 patients with pancreatic ductal disruption and pancreatic ascites treated with transpapillary pancreatic duct stenting, achieving resolution in all patients at 12 months following stent removal.[32] Subsequently, Bracher and colleagues reported their case series of 8 patients with PD disruption and pancreatic ascites, achieving the resolution of ascites in all 8 cases.[33]

Kozarek and colleagues found that pancreatic duct stent placement was associated with the polymicrobial contamination of the pancreas, although most were asymptomatic.[34] However, in situations whereby the patient exhibits symptoms, and the collection is increasing in size, without necrosis, connected to the pancreatic duct, and not amenable to transmural endoscopic intervention, pancreatic duct stent placement with or without a pancreatic sphincterotomy is effective, particularly when the collection is small (<5–6 cm). The ideal approach in such cases would involve bridging the leak to restore continuity[35,36] although this may not be feasible in cases of complete disruption or pancreatic tail leaks, **Box 3**, **Fig. 4**A–D. In such instances, the proximal end of the stent may be positioned downstream from the leak or could enter the pseudocyst directly. There is a chance that pancreatic stents may induce the scarring of the main pancreatic duct in patients with normal ducts.[37]

Das and colleagues conducted a retrospective study that included 107 patients with pancreatic duct (PD) disruption, the majority of whom suffered from pancreatitis (65%). They were able to successfully place a stent in 96% of patients, and in 45 patients (44%) were able to traverse the disrupted duct to restore continuity. Overall, therapeutic success was achieved in 75% of patients. In multivariate analysis, they found the absence of complete pancreatic duct disruption and acute pancreatitis were independent predictors of successful therapy.[38] Ni J et al.[39] performed a multicenter retrospective study whereby they studied 153 patients with pseudocyst (57) and walled off necrosis (96). They had 3 treatment arms including transmural (39), transpapillary (22) or both (92). Complete and partial disruption of the pancreatic duct were seen in 55 and 29 patients, respectively. They were able to restore continuity of PD with stent in 87% and 55% of patients with partial and complete PD disruption. Patients who received combined therapy had a shorter length of hospital stay and a lower recurrence rate.

In surgical cases involving distal pancreatectomy, a Grade A leak is generally considered a biochemical leak that is self-limited and does not require immediate intervention. However, if the leak persists for more than 3 weeks and progresses to a Grade B, endoscopic intervention becomes necessary. This intervention often involves transpapillary stenting, with or without sphincterotomy, and may also include transmural drainage, depending on the specific circumstances.[31,40] Frozanpor and colleagues reported their randomized controlled trial evaluating the effect of prophylactic pancreatic stenting following distal pancreatectomy (DP). They randomized 58 patients to either DP with or without prophylactic stent and found that clinically significant pancreatic fistulas (ISGPF Grade B or C) occurred in 22.2% versus 42.3% in the DP and DP + stent groups, respectively.[41] This trial demonstrated that prophylactic stenting did not reduce the rate of pancreatic fistula following distal pancreatectomy. Sahakian and colleagues reported a case of the use of a metallic coil plus N-butyl-2-cyanoacrylate for closure of a PD leak that occurred following distal pancreatectomy. Standard treatments had failed, and this technique resulted in clinical resolution within 7 days with no adverse events.[42]

Box 3
Case study 2

A 37-year-old female with a history of chronic pancreatitis due to alcohol abuse presented with new-onset ascites, without clinical or imaging findings suggestive of advanced liver disease. She underwent a diagnostic paracentesis, which showed a protein level of 2.4 g/dL, albumin level of 1.9 g/dL, amylase level of 4427 units/L, total bilirubin level of 0.9 mg/dL, and triglyceride level of 17 mg/dL, with a total serum albumin of 1.8 g/dL. This revealed a Serum Ascites Albumin Gradient (SAAG) 1.0. Imaging, including MRI, showed worsening fluid collection and ascites, with the presence of a 3 by 3 cm fluid collection at the pancreas body and upstream pancreatic duct dilation. Due to the worsening ascites and fluid collection, the patient underwent therapeutic Endoscopic Retrograde Pancreatography for the treatment of a pancreatic duct leak (see **Fig. 4**A–D).

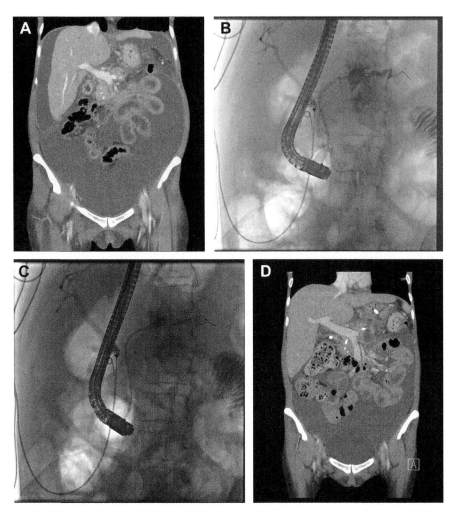

Fig. 4. (*A*) Coronal view of abdominal CT scan revealing a large amount of ascites. (*B*) Fluoroscopy image during endoscopic retrograde pancreatography (ERP) revealing a pancreatic duct leak at the body of the pancreas. (*C*) A plastic pancreatic stent traversing the pancreatic duct disruption toward the tail of the pancreas. (*D*) Repeat CT scan performed 7 days after ERP and stent placement revealing a decrease in the amount of ascites with the pancreatic stent in place, bridging the leak.

FISTULA
External Fistula

These fistulas are commonly observed following surgical or percutaneous therapies for chronic pancreatitis or pseudocysts, and they can also occur after pancreatectomy for various reasons. In cases of postpancreatectomy Grade B leaks that persist for more than 3 weeks, endoscopic intervention is typically indicated, often involving transpapillary pancreatic duct stenting with or without pancreatic sphincterotomy.[31,40] In those whereby there is a percutaneous drain with persistent high output, success depends on the size of the external drain as compared with the internal stent size.

Strategies such as downsizing, clamping, and eventually removing the external drain after successful endoscopic stent placement can help promote internal drainage and lead to fistula closure.[6] It is worth noting that up to 75% of pancreaticocutaneous fistulas may be effectively treated with endoscopic techniques.[43]

Internal Fistula

If the fistula does not respond to conservative therapy with or without somatostatin analogs, the success of transpapillary drainage is dependent on the location and degree of pancreatic disruption. Tanaka and colleagues reported their case series of 6 patients who underwent transpapillary pancreatic stenting for the treatment of an internal pancreatic fistula,5 of which were located in the body and 1 in the tail. Three patients recovered fully with endoscopic stenting, while 3 required surgery.[44] If the fistula is originating from the head or body of the pancreas, a PD stent covering the fistula is highly effective; however, this method is less effective if the fistula originates from the pancreatic tail.[18,45,46] In a series of 43 patients with pancreatic pleural fistula, ERP with stenting was successful in all patients.[47] ERCP with both pancreatic and biliary stenting have been successful in closing pancreatic biliary fistula.[48] In pancreatic tail fistula, there are case reports of using fibrosealant; however, this approach comes with the risk of blockage of the PD at different levels, in addition to other inherent risks of these agents. If the fistula/leak is upstream from complete blockage, endotherapy is not helpful, including in cases with disconnected duct syndrome, which is discussed in another article.

Although most of the upper GI and pancreatic pleural fistula close after sphincterotomy with or without the drainage or debridement of the collection,[20,47,49] however, colonic fistula are more likely to require surgical intervention.[14,20,50]

Cases of chronic pancreatitis present with recurrent acute pancreatitis (RAP) and a fluid collection, likely due to stricture or stones, may need transpapillary intervention.

Adverse Events

Endoscopic therapy in the form of pancreatic duct stenting is generally safe and effective. A thorough review of cross-sectional imaging and appropriate preparation, including multidisciplinary discussion, may help minimize adverse events (AEs). However, despite a comprehensive preprocedure evaluation, AEs may occur. The most common of these is post-ERCP pancreatitis.[10] Rates of pancreatitis range between 10% and 50%, particularly if pancreatic stenting is not achieved despite multiple maneuvers in the duct.[10] The placement of a pancreatic duct stent does lower the risk of pancreatitis, as does the administration of rectal indomethacin.[51,52] Other AEs following ERCP include: bleeding, perforation, anesthetic complications, aspiration, and biliary injury.

SUMMARY

Patients with pancreatic duct leaks and fistulas are best managed by a multidisciplinary team including gastroenterologists, interventional radiologists, and pancreaticobiliary surgeons. Most leaks are able to be managed through either endoscopic therapy or interventional radiologic-guided procedures. Once leaks have failed conservative management, ERP with transpapillary stenting is the mainstay of treatment and the next step in the management in the absence of a disconnected duct. Pancreatic endotherapy will continue to evolve to improve outcomes for patients with pancreatic duct leaks and fistulas.

CLINICS CARE POINTS

Pearls:
- Contrast enhanced CT scan is helpful for the initial evaluation of pancreatic leak/fistula.
- MRCP ± Secretin is more sensitive than a CT scan to delineate pancreatic duct disruption and help as a road map for endotherapy and predict response.
- Acute onset leaks are mostly self-limited and improve over time.
- Intervention through ERP is very effective in persistent leak from partial to complete pancreatic duct disruption.
- In selected cases, ERP with intervention needs to be combined with transmural drainage of the collection.

Pitfalls
- Intervention through ERP may not be as effective in pancreatic tail fistula.
- Complete pancreatic duct disruption is less amenable to endotherapy.
- Fistula arising from a disconnected pancreatic duct are not amenable to transpapillary drainage.

DISCLOSURES

H. Razjouyan has no disclosures. J.L. Maranki is a consultant for Boston Scientific Corp.

REFERENCES

1. Mutignani M, Dokas S, Tringali A, et al. Pancreatic Leaks and Fistulae: An Endoscopy-Oriented Classification. Dig Dis Sci 2017;62(10):2648–57.
2. Kozarek RA. Endoscopic therapy of complete and partial pancreatic duct disruptions. Gastrointest Endosc Clin N Am 1998;8(1):39–53.
3. Balthazar EJ, Robinson DL, Megibow AJ, et al. Acute pancreatitis: value of CT in establishing prognosis. Radiology 1990;174(2):331–6.
4. Baron TH, Morgan DE. Acute necrotizing pancreatitis. N Engl J Med 1999; 340(18):1412–7.
5. Fielding GA, McLatchie GR, Wilson C, et al. Acute pancreatitis and pancreatic fistula formation. Br J Surg 1989;76(11):1126–8.
6. Law R, Baron T. Endoscopic treatment of pancreatic disease. Gastrointestinal and liver disease 2020;1.
7. Allen PJ. Pasireotide for postoperative pancreatic fistula. N Engl J Med 2014; 371(9):875–6.
8. Kao LS, Bulger EM, Parks DL, et al. Predictors of morbidity after traumatic pancreatic injury. J Trauma 2003;55(5):898–905.
9. Sealock RJ, Othman M, Das K. Endoscopic Diagnosis and Management of Gastrointestinal Trauma. Clin Gastroenterol Hepatol 2021;19(1):14–23.
10. Larsen M, Kozarek R. Management of pancreatic ductal leaks and fistulae. J Gastroenterol Hepatol 2014;29(7):1360–70.
11. Morgan KA, Adams DB. Management of internal and external pancreatic fistulas. Surg Clin North Am 2007;87(6):1503–13.
12. Singh A, Aggarwal M, Garg R, et al. Spontaneous Internal Pancreatic Fistulae Complicating Acute Pancreatitis. Am J Gastroenterol 2021;116(7):1381–6.
13. Tsiotos GG, Smith CD, Sarr MG. Incidence and management of pancreatic and enteric fistulas after surgical management of severe necrotizing pancreatitis. Arch Surg 1995;130(1):48–52.

14. Kochhar R, Jain K, Gupta V, et al. Fistulization in the GI tract in acute pancreatitis. Gastrointest Endosc 2012;75(2):436–40.

15. Uomo G, Molino D, Visconti M, et al. The incidence of main pancreatic duct disruption in severe biliary pancreatitis. Am J Surg 1998;176(1):49–52.

16. Jang JW, Kim MH, Oh D, et al. Factors and outcomes associated with pancreatic duct disruption in patients with acute necrotizing pancreatitis. Pancreatology 2016;16(6):958–65.

17. Machado NO. Pancreaticopleural fistula: revisited. Diagn Ther Endosc 2012; 2012:815476.

18. Sasturkar SV, Gupta S, Thapar S, et al. Endoscopic management of pleural effusion caused by a pancreatic pleural fistula. J Postgrad Med 2020;66(4):206–8.

19. Frakes JT. Biliary pancreatitis: a review. Emphasizing appropriate endoscopic intervention. J Clin Gastroenterol 1999;28(2):97–109.

20. Jiang W, Tong Z, Yang D, et al. Gastrointestinal Fistulas in Acute Pancreatitis With Infected Pancreatic or Peripancreatic Necrosis: A 4-Year Single-Center Experience. Medicine (Baltim) 2016;95(14):e3318.

21. Aswani Y, Hira P. Pancreaticopleural fistula: a review. JOP 2015;16(1):90–4.

22. Kozarek RA. Pancreatic Duct Leaks and Pseudocysts. In: Ginsberg GG, Gostout CJ, Kochman ML, Norton ID, editors. Clinical Gastrointestinal Endoscopy. Second Edition. Philadelphia, PA: W.B. Saunders; 2012. p. 692–705.

23. De Waele JJ, Delrue L, Hoste EA, et al. Extrapancreatic inflammation on abdominal computed tomography as an early predictor of disease severity in acute pancreatitis: evaluation of a new scoring system. Pancreas 2007;34(2):185–90.

24. Bollen TL, Singh VK, Maurer R, et al. A comparative evaluation of radiologic and clinical scoring systems in the early prediction of severity in acute pancreatitis. Am J Gastroenterol 2012;107(4):612–9.

25. Gupta A, Stuhlfaut JW, Fleming KW, et al. Blunt trauma of the pancreas and biliary tract: a multimodality imaging approach to diagnosis. Radiographics 2004;24(5): 1381–95.

26. Mortele KJ, Wiesner W, Intriere L, et al. A modified CT severity index for evaluating acute pancreatitis: improved correlation with patient outcome. AJR Am J Roentgenol 2004;183(5):1261–5.

27. Fulcher AS, Turner MA, Yelon JA, et al. Magnetic resonance cholangiopancreatography (MRCP) in the assessment of pancreatic duct trauma and its sequelae: preliminary findings. J Trauma 2000;48(6):1001–7.

28. Gillams AR, Kurzawinski T, Lees WR. Diagnosis of duct disruption and assessment of pancreatic leak with dynamic secretin-stimulated MR cholangiopancreatography. AJR Am J Roentgenol 2006;186(2):499–506.

29. Takishima T, Hirata M, Kataoka Y, et al. Pancreatographic classification of pancreatic ductal injuries caused by blunt injury to the pancreas. J Trauma 2000;48(4): 745–51 [discussion 751-2].

30. Villena V, Pérez V, Pozo F, et al. Amylase levels in pleural effusions: a consecutive unselected series of 841 patients. Chest 2002;121(2):470–4.

31. Bassi C, Marchegiani G, Dervenis C, et al. The 2016 update of the International Study Group (ISGPS) definition and grading of postoperative pancreatic fistula: 11 Years After. Surgery 2017;161(3):584–91.

32. Kozarek RA, Jiranek GC, Traverso LW. Endoscopic treatment of pancreatic ascites. Am J Surg 1994;168(3):223–6.

33. Bracher GA, Manocha AP, DeBanto JR, et al. Endoscopic pancreatic duct stenting to treat pancreatic ascites. Gastrointest Endosc 1999;49(6):710–5.

34. Kozarek RA, Traverso LW. Pancreatic fistulas: etiology, consequences, and treatment. Gastroenterol 1996;4(4):238–44.
35. Telford JJ, Farrell JJ, Saltzman JR, et al. Pancreatic stent placement for duct disruption. Gastrointest Endosc 2002;56(1):18–24.
36. Varadarajulu S, Noone TC, Tutuian R, et al. Predictors of outcome in pancreatic duct disruption managed by endoscopic transpapillary stent placement. Gastrointest Endosc 2005;61(4):568–75.
37. Rashdan A, Fogel EL, McHenry L, et al. Improved stent characteristics for prophylaxis of post-ERCP pancreatitis. Clin Gastroenterol Hepatol 2004;2(4):322–9.
38. Das R, Papachristou GI, Slivka A, et al. Endotherapy is effective for pancreatic ductal disruption: A dual center experience. Pancreatology 2016;16(2):278–83.
39. Ni J, Peng K, Yu L, et al. Transpapillary Stenting Improves Treatment Outcomes in Patients Undergoing Endoscopic Transmural Drainage of Ductal Disruption-Associated Pancreatic Fluid Collections. Am J Gastroenterol 2023;118(6): 972–82.
40. Coté GA. Treatment of postoperative pancreatic fluid collections. Gastrointest Endosc 2020;91(5):1092–4.
41. Frozanpor F, Lundell L, Segersvärd R, et al. The effect of prophylactic transpapillary pancreatic stent insertion on clinically significant leak rate following distal pancreatectomy: results of a prospective controlled clinical trial. Ann Surg 2012;255(6):1032–6.
42. Sahakian AB, Jayaram P, Marx MV, et al. Metallic coil and N-butyl-2-cyanoacrylate for closure of pancreatic duct leak (with video). Gastrointest Endosc 2018; 87(4):1122–5.
43. Malleo G, Pulvirenti A, Marchegiani G, et al. Diagnosis and management of postoperative pancreatic fistula. Langenbeck's Arch Surg 2014;399(7):801–10.
44. Tanaka T, Kuroki T, Kitasato A, et al. Endoscopic transpapillary pancreatic stenting for internal pancreatic fistula with the disruption of the pancreatic ductal system. Pancreatology 2013;13(6):621–4.
45. Boerma D, Rauws EA, van Gulik TM, et al. Endoscopic stent placement for pancreaticocutaneous fistula after surgical drainage of the pancreas. Br J Surg 2000; 87(11):1506–9.
46. Lau ST, Simchuk EJ, Kozarek RA, et al. A pancreatic ductal leak should be sought to direct treatment in patients with acute pancreatitis. Am J Surg 2001;181(5): 411–5.
47. Kord Valeshabad A, Acostamadiedo J, Xiao L, et al. Pancreaticopleural Fistula: A Review of Imaging Diagnosis and Early Endoscopic Intervention. Case Rep Gastrointest Med 2018;2018:7589451.
48. Carrere C, Heyries L, Barthet M, et al. Biliopancreatic fistulas complicating pancreatic pseudocysts: a report of three cases demonstrated by endoscopic retrograde cholangiopancreatography. Endoscopy 2001;33(1):91–4.
49. Halttunen J, Weckman L, Kemppainen E, et al. The endoscopic management of pancreatic fistulas. Surg Endosc 2005;19(4):559–62.
50. Mohamed SR, Siriwardena AK. Understanding the colonic complications of pancreatitis. Pancreatology 2008;8(2):153–8.
51. Tarnasky PR, Palesch YY, Cunningham JT, et al. Pancreatic stenting prevents pancreatitis after biliary sphincterotomy in patients with sphincter of Oddi dysfunction. Gastroenterology 1998;115(6):1518–24.
52. Elmunzer BJ, Scheiman JM, Lehman GA, et al. A randomized trial of rectal indomethacin to prevent post-ERCP pancreatitis. N Engl J Med 2012;366(15): 1414–22.

Pancreatoscopy-Guided Endotherapies for Pancreatic Diseases

Yuri Hanada, MD[a], Raj J. Shah, MD, MASGE, AGAF, FACG[b],*

KEYWORDS

- Pancreatoscopy • Cholangioscopy • Intraductal papillary mucinous neoplasm
- Pancreatic duct stone • Dilated pancreatic duct • Lithotripsy
- Pancreatic duct stricture • Stricturoplasty

KEY POINTS

- Per-oral pancreatoscopy (POP) allows for the performance of pancreatic duct interventions under direct visualization and assists with pancreas preservation.
- POP is a pancreas-preserving modality that has an emerging role in the accurate diagnosis, risk stratification, and disease extent determination of suspected and established main duct intraductal papillary mucinous neoplasms (IPMNs). It may emerge as a technique for laser ablation of symptomatic mucin-secreting IPMNs in medically inoperable or surgically unresectable patients.
- POP-guided endotherapies for obstructive chronic pancreatitis—including intraductal lithotripsy and laser stricturoplasty—are emerging and appear effective.
- POP and the growing armamentarium of device-specific accessories allows for effective foreign body and stone fragment removal from the pancreatic duct.
- A command of therapeutic pancreatic endoscopic retrograde pancreatography is required prior to embarking on an endoscopic practice that includes POP.

 Video content accompanies this article at http://www.giendo.theclinics.com.

INTRODUCTION

Per-oral pancreatoscopy (POP) entails passage of a miniature catheter-based disposable endoscope through the working channel of a duodenoscope as an adjunct to endoscopic retrograde pancreatography (ERP) to allow access to and directly visualize the pancreatic duct. By allowing inspection of the duct and any associated

a Division of Gastroenterology, Hennepin Healthcare, 701 Park Avenue, Mail Code O1, Minneapolis, MN 55415, USA; b Division of Gastroenterology and Hepatology, University of Colorado Anschutz Medical Campus, 1635 Aurora Court, Mail Stop F 735, Aurora, CO 80045, USA
* Corresponding author.
E-mail address: Raj.Shah@cuanschutz.edu

Gastrointest Endoscopy Clin N Am 34 (2024) 417–431
https://doi.org/10.1016/j.giec.2024.02.007
1052-5157/24/© 2024 Elsevier Inc. All rights reserved.

pathology, POP can overcome a number of current diagnostic and therapeutic limitations of advanced radiographic pancreatic imaging and standard ERP techniques, respectively. Established POP-guided interventions include the detection and assessment of the extent of main duct intraductal papillary mucinous neoplasms (IPMNs) and intraductal lithotripsy of difficult pancreatic duct stones.[1-5] This review will also discuss the emerging POP-guided techniques of laser stricturoplasty, neoplasia ablation, and foreign body removal.[6-8]

PROCEDURE PREPARATION
Sedation

General anesthesia is recommended due to the use of intraductal saline irrigation during POP, which can result in pooling of fluid within the upper gastrointestinal tract and increase risk for aspiration.[1]

Patient Positioning

Semi-prone positioning is our preference to maximize ergonomics during potentially prolonged procedures, duodenoscope stability for the initial insertion of the pancreatoscope, and maintenance of the pancreatoscope position throughout the duration of the case.

Equipment

Pancreatoscopy is primarily performed using systems that were initially designed for cholangioscopy, as outlined in the American Society for Gastrointestinal Endoscopy Technology Committee Status Evaluation Report.[2] Currently, in the United States, only the catheter-based, single-operator SpyGlass DS II System (Boston Scientific, Marlborough, MA, USA) is approved by the Food and Drug Administration (FDA) for pancreatic duct visualization. The system is a 10.5-Fr catheter with a tip capable of 4-way deflection via 2 control wheels, a 1.2 mm working channel, and independent irrigation channels.[1] The most current generation of this system, released in 2018, contains a complementary metal-oxide semiconductor chip for high dynamic range image processing, as well as adjusted lighting to reduce the incidence of light flare.[9]

GENERAL TECHNIQUE

Pancreatoscopy is completed within the context of ERP. A strong command of ERP is required prior to incorporating pancreatoscopy into one's practice due to the cognitive skills needed to appropriately identify cases and pathology, as well as technical skills needed to safely manage the pancreatoscope and accessories throughout the case and any potential adverse events (AEs). After pancreatic cannulation is achieved with standard ERP devices, a guidewire is advanced to the maximal extent of the main pancreatic duct depending on tortuosity and pathology. Pancreatic sphincterotomy is then performed to allow introduction of the pancreatoscope into the duct, unless the pancreatic orifice is patulous enough for easy entry without intervention. Judicious sterile saline irrigation is recommended to reduce the theoretic risk of increased intraparenchymal pressure and subsequent post-procedural pancreatitis or pain flare-ups of chronic pancreatitis.[5] Dilation of downstream strictures with a minimum balloon diameter of 4 mm may be required to ensure successful advancement of the 10-Fr pancreatoscope.[1]

Long guidewires, generally 450 cm in length and 0.025″ or 0.035″ in diameter, allow for "back-end" guidewire tension control during introduction of the pancreatoscope over the guidewire through the duodenoscope working channel and subsequently into the duct. Short-wire access is also possible, and preferred by the authors, given ease-of-use with staff and provided that the elevator is used to secure the wire during POP advancement while the wire is "floated." The angle of pancreatic duct cannulation with the pancreatoscope is typically favorable as compared to the bile duct due to the oblique angulation. However, if there is difficulty with the initial advancement, the 2 control wheels of the pancreatoscope can be used to deflect the tip into a more appropriate direction. The control wheels, which can lock, are subsequently used to aid in controlled navigation through the duct. The guidewire is then removed prior to inspection on withdrawal to free the working channel for device passage, as necessary.[1]

Occasionally, accessory devices are unable to pass through the working channel of the pancreatoscope due to angulation of the system as it exits from the duodenoscope through the papilla. In these cases, withdrawing the pancreatoscope to the downstream pancreatic duct, or alternatively advancing it further up the duct, can allow for subsequent passage of the accessory through and out of the working channel. If the POP dials were locked to facilitate inspection, ensure that the dials are unlocked if there is difficulty with advancing devices out of the working channel. For acute angulations and while approaching pathology in the downstream duct, a reasonable option is withdrawing the pancreatoscope from the duct into the duodenal lumen to reduce the angulation for accessory passage and advancing the accessory with minimal tip protrusion during free-hand cannulation.

INDICATIONS AND APPROACH
Assessment and Management of Intraductal Papillary Mucinous Neoplasms

IPMNs are pancreatic cystic lesions of ductal epithelium origin with variable malignant potential.[4] The risk of dysplasia and malignant transformation, as well as the incidence of harboring coexisting invasive carcinoma at diagnosis, is significantly higher for IPMNs involving the main pancreatic duct, as compared to IPMNs of the side branch or mixed subtypes.[4,10]

Accurate diagnosis, risk stratification, and disease extent determination, which in turn guide management decisions that can range from repeat imaging to complex surgical resection and reconstruction, currently rely on pancreatic cross-sectional imaging and endoscopic ultrasound with cystic fluid analysis. However, these investigative modes remain suboptimal in the setting of dilated pancreatic ducts and can be associated with misclassification errors due to poor correlation between imaging and histopathologic diagnosis given a paucity of epithelial cells during sampling and limited sensitivity in differentiating benign versus malignant early lesions.[3,11] Both undertreatment, with potential for disease progression, and overtreatment, with unnecessary loss of pancreatic parenchyma, can result in serious consequences, underlining the importance of improving diagnostic, risk stratification, and disease extent identification capabilities.

Over the past few decades, POP has played a growing role in the assessment and management of IPMNs. POP advantageously allows for direct visualization of IPMN-associated ductal mucosal changes, specifically those that correspond with malignancy. Targeted biopsies with increased diagnostic yield can be obtained via POP, particularly in cases where standard-of-care endoscopic ultrasound with fine needle aspiration provides inconclusive results regarding the presence of dysplasia or malignancy.[10,12] Importantly, direct visualization of IPMNs via POP confers the ability to significantly inform surgical management through accurate, rather than estimated, mapping of disease extent, with the primary goal of achieving adequate resection with maximal preservation of pancreatic parenchyma.[13] Concern for disease recurrence centers on the possible presence of discontinuous, or "skip," IPMN lesions, which have been described in surgical case series at rates of up to 19%, and in some cases, can result in need for reoperation.[14] Conversely, POP can spare patients from total pancreatectomy despite extensive preoperative evaluation indicating need for total pancreatectomy.[13] **Fig. 1** outlines a proposed workflow for incorporating POP in the evaluation and management of main duct IPMNs.

Of note, there have been additional emerging roles for POP in the assessment and management of IPMNs described which have the potential to impact clinical approach. First is the diagnosis of occult IPMNs. In 1 case series, POP identified main duct IPMN in 13 patients with presumed idiopathic chronic calcific pancreatitis with dilated pancreatic duct.[15] For this reason, we recommend considering POP if the pancreatic duct is dilated above 5 mm during the evaluation of patients who do not have an identifiable etiology for chronic calcific pancreatitis (**Fig. 2**).

A second utilization of POP in the setting of IPMNs is neoplasia ablation. Cholangioscopy with argon plasma coagulation ablation of a neoplastic biliary lesion analogous to

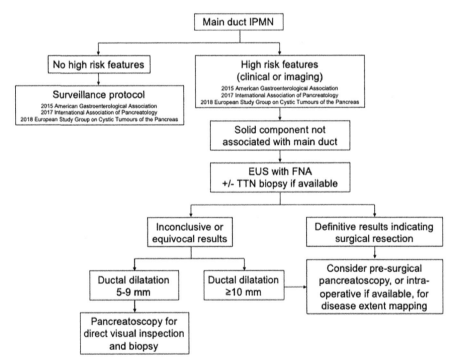

Fig. 1. Role of pancreatoscopy for the evaluation of main duct intraductal papillary mucinous neoplasms. A proposed workflow for the use of pancreatoscopy in the management of main duct IPMNs. The main utility of pancreatoscopy in the preoperative or intraoperative setting is to avoid under-resection as can occur with skip lesions, while ensuring minimal but adequate resection for maximal preservation of pancreatic parenchyma. For all patients with diagnosed main duct IPMNs, referral to a comprehensive multidisciplinary pancreas lesion clinic is recommended if available. This proposed workflow is based on the assumption that the patient has been deemed surgically appropriate. EUS, endoscopic ultrasound; FNA, fine needle aspiration; IPMN, intraductal papillary mucinous neoplasm; TTN, through-the-needle.

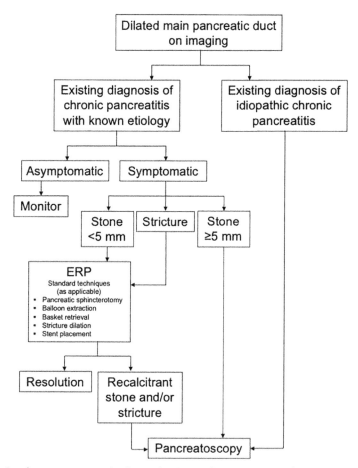

Fig. 2. Role of pancreatoscopy in the evaluation and management of main pancreatic duct dilatation. A proposed algorithm for the use of pancreatoscopy in the evaluation and management of main pancreatic duct dilatation. From a therapeutic standpoint, pancreatoscopy should be considered when (1) stones ≥5 mm are identified due to low likelihood of successful clearance with standard techniques, (2) electrohydraulic or laser lithotripsy are needed to address recalcitrant stones, or (3) laser stricturoplasty is needed to address recalcitrant stricture. Strictures are often present downstream to large stones and require treatment prior to attempting pancreatoscopy-guided lithotripsy to ensure the ability of the duct to accommodate the pancreatoscope. Diagnostically, pancreatoscopy may identify occult main duct intraductal papillary mucinous neoplasms in patients with previously presumed idiopathic chronic pancreatitis and associated pancreatic duct dilatation. ERP, endoscopic retrograde pancreatography.

IPMN has previously been described.[16] In this case, the patient was deemed surgical unfit, but due to recurrent bouts of cholangitis, was offered ablative therapy with the goal of reducing obstructing mucin production. Similar ablative therapy has also been described to address symptomatic IPMNs of the pancreas.[7,17] In 1 case, a patient with recurrent acute pancreatitis of undetermined etiology superimposed on chronic pancreatitis related to pancreas divisum underwent standard minor papilla sphincterotomy and upsizing of therapeutic pancreatic stents to no effect. POP was therefore performed to elucidate the etiology and successfully identified IPMN-like mucosal changes in a side branch, with pathology confirming IPMN with low-grade dysplasia. Notably, in this case, cross-sectional imaging failed to identify the presence of side branch IPMNs. Due to poor surgical candidacy and poor response to conventional measures, laser-guided ablation of the lesion to reduce ductal obstruction from mucin production was successfully performed, with no subsequent episodes of acute pancreatitis thereafter now at 45 months of follow-up. In this case, a Holmium laser was used under soft tissue settings, as described in the section titled, "Laser Stricturoplasty."

The general technique for POP evaluation of IPMN is as follows. After cannulation of the pancreatic duct with the pancreatoscope is achieved, the pancreatoscope is advanced to the level of the pancreas tail. As the pancreatoscope is withdrawn from the tail toward the ampulla, the duct is judiciously immersed in normal saline solution to permit clear intraductal visualization and the mucosa is carefully inspected. In the case of a heavy mucin burden within the duct, we encourage sweeping of as much mucin as possible with a stone extraction balloon prior to POP insertion. Further, this is the scenario in which a higher force of saline irrigation may be required to assure optimal visualization. We obtain spot films of the pancreatoscope at lesional areas that may help discussions with our surgical colleagues regarding the planned extent of resection.

Benign and malignant IPMNs can often be differentiated based on morphologic appearance on POP utilizing Hara's classification, but reliance on histologic samples remains.[18] Lesions with granular mucosa (type 1) or fish-egg–like protrusions without visible vascularity (type 2) are associated with benign hyperplastic or adenomatous growth in 100% of cases, whereas lesions with fish-egg–like protrusions with visible vascularity (type 3), villous protrusions (type 4), or vegetative protrusions (type 5) are associated with carcinoma in situ or invasive carcinoma in 89%, 92%, and 91% of cases, respectively.[18] Narrow band imaging, if using an image-enhanced capable POP system, can further increase visibility of mucosal abnormalities and capillary vessels.[19–21]

Once mucosal inspection has been completed, biopsies can be obtained under direct visualization for gold standard tissue diagnosis. The SpyGlass DS II System includes 2 types of forceps devices, termed SpyBite Biopsy Forceps and SpyBite MAX, with the latter representing an updated larger capacity design with additional gripping teeth and drainage holes to decrease sample contamination.[22] The forceps device exits the pancreatoscope in the 6 o'clock orientation and maintains a level of flexibility combined with pushability to allow for a tangential approach to the target area. As the jaws of the forceps close around the tissue target, gentle constant forward pressure against the tissue should be maintained in an attempt to maximize tissue within the cup of the closed forceps and to 'shear' the tissue. A minimum of 3 passes (we prefer obtaining 6 pieces of tissue) is recommended by the manufacturer to ensure diagnostically acceptable samples.

Lithotripsy

Up to 90% of patients with chronic pancreatitis may develop pancreatic duct stones, which can result in significant symptomatic burden.[23] In cases of obstructing calculi, the primary goal of endotherapy is pain relief via stone removal, with consequent duct decompression and mitigation of stone-induced ductal hypertension.[24] Either extracorporeal shock wave lithotripsy (ESWL) or POP-guided intervention for obstructing stones is preferred over surgical resection or drainage given the associated morbidity with loss of pancreatic parenchyma, as well as rates of lack of pain resolution and/or recurrence postoperatively.[25–28]

Conventional treatment options for pancreatic duct stone removal include ERP with pancreatic sphincterotomy, dilation of downstream strictures, balloon sweep stone extraction, and/or basket stone retrieval.[29] Given the mechanisms by which standard ERP techniques accomplish removal, these options are typically limited to non-impacted stones and those smaller than 5 mm in diameter located in the downstream pancreatic duct.[30] Often, however, downstream strictures prevent the removal of even small and mobile stones. For stones larger than 5 mm, data and guidelines support the use of ESWL with or without subsequent ERP due to high effectiveness at stone fragmentation.[31,32] However, ESWL is limited in its ability to address radiolucent stones, multiple stones, stones in patients with high body mass indices, or those overlying the spine which may be difficult to visualize for targeting.[5,29] ESWL also cannot simultaneously address downstream pancreatic duct strictures which may result in ineffective clearance of stone fragments and are associated with high rates of stone recurrence.[5,29,33] Lastly, ESWL for pancreatic stone therapy is not yet widely available in the United States.[32]

POP-guided lithotripsy has emerged as an attractive and efficient alternative for the treatment of obstructing pancreatic duct stones because it allows for stone fragmentation, fragment removal, and stricture treatment if needed within the same procedural session.[5] Additionally, the ability to accurately adjust the application of shock waves with a directed probe increases effectiveness while potentially decreasing associated complications such as pancreatic duct wall injury.[34]

Intraductal lithotripsy is accomplished via electrohydraulic or laser therapy as the duct is immersed in normal saline solution to permit clear intraductal visualization and to transmit the shock wave. The choice of either depends on institutional equipment availability and provider preference, though only laser is FDA-approved for pancreatic duct stone lithotripsy. The authors believe laser lithotripsy is the preferred modality for pancreatic duct stones given their density compared to biliary stones. Electrohydraulic lithotripsy (EHL) utilizes electrodes to generate high-amplitude hydraulic pressure waves, whereas laser lithotripsy uses laser energy pulses through a focused beam to generate a mechanical shock wave.[35] After cannulation of the pancreatic duct with the pancreatoscope is achieved, the pancreatoscope is advanced to the level of the stone under direct visualization. With EHL, an EHL probe (AUTOLITH, Northgate Technologies, Inc., Elgin, Illinois, USA) is advanced through the working channel of the pancreatoscope into the duct and generally placed about 1 mm from the stone; occasionally, stone contact is required for effective fragmentation. EHL is then performed under power settings that can be adjusted based on the responsiveness of the stone; generally, an initial setting of medium power and 10 shots per second is reasonable.[5,36] Higher power may reduce the durability of the probe. The stone fragments can be flushed out with irrigation and extracted following withdrawal of the EHL probe and pancreatoscope, using standard balloon sweep stone extraction and/or basket stone retrieval. Often, we inform patients that small fragments can be retained in side branches or upstream to existing stenoses and subsequent ERP may be required for ductal clearance. The SpyGlass Retrieval Basket (Boston Scientific, Inc) can also be used to capture stone fragments under direct visualization along with the MicroCatch catheter (MTW Endoskopie Manufaktur, Dusseldorf, Germany).[37]

For laser lithotripsy, the use of holmium laser (VersaPulse PowerSuite, Lumenis Ltd., San Jose, California, USA; VersaPulse PowerSuite, New Star Lasers, Roseville, California, USA) has been described.[38] A 200-μm to 365-μm laser fiber is advanced into the duct and aimed toward the stone without directly touching, at a distance of 1 mm. We prefer the 272-μm fiber which passes more easily through the 1.2-mm working channel and permits better tip deflection of the pancreatoscope for stone targeting compared to the larger fiber. Contact of the laser fiber to the stone may bore a hole in the stone but is sometimes necessary in order to initiate fragmentation of very dense stones. Once fragmentation is initiated, laser applications targeting the stone periphery can then be performed. The laser is applied at suggested settings of frequency between 8 to 14 Hz, energy between 1 to 10.5 J, and power between 5 to 10 W, though we have found the need to increase the power when managing difficult stones.[38] Additional advantages to laser are the ability to continue the use of the same fiber throughout the procedure duration by trimming the sheath if and when glass fiber breakage occurs and to adjust retropulsion settings to reduce upstream migration of stone fragments during attempts to further decrease fragment size for easier extraction.[39]

Fig. 2 outlines a proposed algorithm for use of POP in the management of pancreatic duct stones.

Laser Stricturoplasty

Approximately 20% of patients with chronic pancreatitis develop main pancreatic duct strictures.[6,24] As with ductal calculi, the primary goal of stricture treatment is to relieve symptoms by reducing ductal hypertension.[24] Conventional endoscopic management strategy involves multiple ERP sessions over several months during which plastic stents of increasing diameter, multiple plastic stents side-by-side, or fully covered metal stents are placed into the duct spanning the stricture.[6,24] However, a proportion of patients will develop refractory strictures, defined as persistent or relapse of stricture despite minimum 1 year of stenting, that render them "stent-dependent."[6] An alternative definition includes early relapse of symptomatic stenosis following a stent-free trial. In some challenging chronic pancreatitis cases, obstructing calculi with associated downstream strictures may prevent passage of guidewires, optimal pre-POP stricture dilation, or passage of catheter-based devices.[40]

POP may overcome the limitations of standard ERP techniques by offering the ability to directly visualize strictures for the dissection of obstructing fibrotic mucosa and restore or improve ductal patency to permit pancreatoscope position to target obstructing calculi within the same procedural session.[7,40]

The use of holmium soft tissue settings (Litho, Quanta System, Samarate, Italy) and thulium (Cyber TM, Quanta System, Samarate, Italy) lasers has been described.[6,7,40] Thulium is particularly recommended for stricturoplasty and neoplastic ablation, as previously described, due to continuous but shallower tissue penetration depth of up to 0.25 mm and more cut versus coagulation effect.[6,41] After cannulation of the pancreatic duct with the pancreatoscope is achieved, a 200-μm to 272-μm laser fiber (International Medical Lasers, Tualatin, Oregon, USA; Lumenis Ltd, San Jose, California, USA; New Star Lasers, Roseville, California, USA) is advanced to the target area, which is immersed in normal saline solution to permit clear intraductal visualization. Concise and gentle strokes are then used to apply bursts of laser energy along the concentric band of strictured tissue from a distal to proximal of the pancreatoscope approach.[6] Cuts in the fibrotic tissue are made in 3 out of 4 quadrant fashion as the 12 o'clock position may be difficult to access due to the exit location of the laser fiber from the pancreatoscope in the 6 o'clock orientation.[6,40] Lower power settings are suggested for stricturoplasty as compared to lithotripsy, such as a frequency of 8 to 10 Hz, energy of 0.5 J, and power of 5 to 8 W.[6] Care should be exercised in limiting dissection to the minimum amount necessary to achieve the goal of either improving lumen patency or ability to target stones and avoid excessive laser application. The technique of stricturoplasty generally includes adjunctive balloon dilation following laser application to optimize lumen patency. Therapeutic pancreatic stent placement is then performed, with the stent left in place until reassessment of the stricture and ductal patency on routine follow-up ERP.[40] Refer to Video 1 for a demonstration of laser stricturoplasty and lithotripsy.

Fig. 2 outlines a proposed algorithm for use of POP in the management of pancreatic duct strictures.

Foreign Body Removal

Data suggest that migration of therapeutic pancreatic stents upstream into the pancreatic duct occurs in approximately 5% of cases on follow-up.[42] While these stents can be endoscopically removed 78% to 100% of the time using standard instruments such as occlusion balloon catheters, biopsy forceps, baskets, and snares, retrieval can be technically challenging due to narrower ductal anatomy than the biliary tree, associated strictures, stent-associated changes, and migration of fractured stents to the genu or further upstream. Failure of stent retrieval can result in pancreatitis, pancreatic abscess, ductal disruption, ductal occlusion, and eventual need for surgical intervention.[43,44]

POP advantageously allows for direct visualization of foreign bodies within the pancreatic duct for targeted removal. The first description of pancreatoscopy-guided removal of a foreign body involved extraction of a stent fragment that had fractured in the pancreatic body during attempted removal using standard techniques due to stone-related impaction and fibrosis encasing the stent fragment.[7] Laser lithotripsy was performed over multiple sessions to gradually reduce stone burden but eventually laser stricturoplasty was required to dissect and ablate surrounding fibrotic tissue to improve ductal visualization and identify the fragmented stent. Eventually, guidewire advancement under direct visualization through the lumen of the pancreatic stent fragment was successful, followed by device exchange for a Soehendra stent retriever to achieve successful stent removal.[7] The patient was ultimately spared from surgical resection, which would have likely required extended pancreatic tail resection due to the location of the foreign body.

The current SpyGlass DS II System includes devices that can be used, as with the SpyBite Forceps and SpyGlass Retrieval Basket, or are specifically designed, as with the SpyGlass Retrieval Snare, to capture and remove foreign bodies. Published accounts describe successful removal of migrated pancreatic stents using the available SpyGlass accessories, which may require a staged approach of sequential transpapillary stent upsizing to accommodate the pancreatoscope in less dilated downstream ducts prior to removal attempts.[7,8,45] In 2 published cases, after cannulation of the pancreatic duct with the pancreatoscope, a snare was successfully introduced through the pancreatoscope into the pancreatic duct lumen and used to ensnare the downstream portion of the stent, after which the pancreatoscope and ensnared stent were removed in tandem from the pancreatic duct into the duodenal lumen (Video 2).[8,45] One of these cases additionally utilized a retrieval basket and forceps to successfully remove additional fragments of stent material.[45]

OUTCOMES
Assessment and Management of Intraductal Papillary Mucinous Neoplasms

POP's utility in the evaluation of main duct IPMNs has been established for nearly 2 decades and historically is the first indication of how POP has been utilized to guide surgical intervention.[3,18,46] A meta-analysis found that POP has consistently high diagnostic accuracy for IPMNs, at an overall rate between 87.5% and 100%.[47] Overall sensitivity has been reported between 64% and 100% and overall specificity between 75% and 100% for the diagnosis of IPMNs.[47]

Using the Hara visual classification scheme of lesion morphology, POP has a sensitivity, specificity, and accuracy of 68%, 87%, and 75%, respectively in differentiating malignant from benign IPMN lesions.[18] POP has also been shown to specifically identify additional high-risk features that were not seen on cross-sectional imaging or endoscopic ultrasound in 42% of patients.[48]

With IPMNs for which surgery is indicated, current standard of care involves partial pancreatic resection with intraoperative frozen section analysis when there is no imaging evidence to support IPMN involvement of the entire main pancreatic duct.[13] This approach assumes, however, that the analyzed section is representative of the remaining duct and parenchyma and no skip lesions are present.[13] Additionally, some centers recommend total pancreatectomy upfront if the pancreatic duct is significantly diffusely dilated or starting with partial central pancreatectomy with further incremental resections based on bilateral margins up to total pancreatectomy, pancreaticoduodenectomy, or extended left pancreatectomy despite the significant morbidity associated with the parenchymal loss of both total and central pancreatectomy procedures.[49,50]

Preoperative POP has proven to be an accurate method of mapping the extent of IPMN lesions, including possible skip lesions and uninvolved regions, along the length of the main pancreatic duct.[10,51] Two prospective studies have demonstrated the ability of POP to inform surgical decision-making in up to approximately 75% of cases, with half of cases requiring more extensive resection and half of cases downstaging to less-extensive resection.[10,51] Moreover, pancreatoscopy in the intraoperative setting has been proposed as a way to provide exacting, "personalized" margins while decreasing the risk of post-ERP pancreatitis due to direct insertion of the pancreatoscope into the pancreatic duct.[10] Intraoperative pancreatoscopy has been shown to change the operative course in 65% of cases, with 67% of those cases requiring extended resection.[13] Results from a large, international, multicenter study on the use of intraoperative pancreatoscopy for patients undergoing resection for main duct IPMNs are awaited.

Lithotripsy

Since the earliest published series, POP-guided lithotripsy has proven to be highly effective.[38,52] A large, multicenter study demonstrated a technical success, or complete stone clearance, rate of 89.9% and clinical success rate, defined as symptomatic improvement or resolution, of 88.4%, with 73.5% of cases requiring only 1 session to achieve technical success.[53] Subsequent meta-analyses support these findings, with overall pooled technical success ranging from 88.1% to 91.2% and pooled clinical success reported at 87.1%.[35,54] Additionally, pancreatoscopy-guided lithotripsy achieves long-term clinical success, defined as lack of symptomatic recurrence attributable to imaging-confirmed intraductal stones, at higher rates compared to historical ESWL data, specifically 63% at median follow-up of 35 months versus 39% at median follow-up of 76.5 months, respectively.[55] As of publication, there is an ongoing multicenter randomized clinical trial (NCT04115826) comparing the efficacy of POP-guided lithotripsy versus ESWL in treating refractory main pancreatic duct stones and achieving duct clearance in chronic pancreatitis patients.[29]

In the cholangioscopy literature, there is strong evidence demonstrating laser lithotripsy as a superior modality versus EHL and ESWL in terms of stone fragmentation and ductal clearance rates.[56] Preliminary survey of the POP-guided lithotripsy literature suggests that laser lithotripsy will statistically outperform EHL in technical success, clinical success, and single session success, as more data become available.[35,53] There is a significant reduction in procedural time when using laser lithotripsy, attributable to the increased ability of laser to fragment denser stones.[53]

Laser Stricturoplasty

In early case series of this technique, laser stricturoplasty for the treatment of refractory pancreaticobiliary strictures resulted in an immediate technical success rate, defined as ability to traverse the stricture with the pancreatoscope immediately after dissection, of 94% and a short-term technical success rate, defined as greater than 90% resolution of the stricture on subsequent pancreatography, of 88%.[6,7] Long-term data on its effectiveness in reducing the need for repeat stenting or other intervention for pain management are awaited.

Adverse Events

Diagnostic and therapeutic pancreatoscopy has a reported pooled AE rate of 12%.[47] Considering that POP may often assist with minimizing or avoiding surgical intervention, the AE rate is considered acceptable. In our experience, patients with chronic pancreatitis are relatively immune to severe post-procedure pancreatitis, especially when a pancreatic duct stent is placed. Post-ERP pancreatitis, which may manifest as a pain flare-up alone requiring an overnight extended recovery stay, is the most common AE and is typically mild.[47] Other usual AEs following ERP include bleeding and perforation.

SUMMARY

Despite advances in ERP technique and devices, the endoscopic management of pancreatic disorders remains challenging due to the underlying pathology and potential ongoing lifestyle contributors such as cigarette smoking. In select cases, POP expands the endoscopist's toolbox by allowing visual diagnosis and performance of targeted pancreatic duct interventions. In particular, POP is an endotherapy that has an emerging role in pancreas preservation for challenging and complex cases for which standard ERP methods are unable to achieve diagnostic and therapeutic success. A command of therapeutic pancreatic ERP is required prior to embarking on an endoscopic practice that includes POP. As experience and comfort with POP increases beyond select referral center practices, further studies validating POP efficacy with long-term follow-up will help to clarify where POP-guided intervention is most beneficial and when or if surgical intervention may be preferred.

CLINICS CARE POINTS

- In patients with main duct intraductal papillary mucinous neoplasm (IPMN) with inconclusive or equivocal sampling results by standard methods despite high risk clinical or imaging features, consider per-oral pancreatoscopy (POP) for direct visualization and biopsy.
- In patients with main duct IPMN proceeding to surgical resection, consider POP either in the pre-surgical or intra-operative setting for disease extent mapping.
- Consider POP for ablation of symptomatic IPMN in patients who are unable to proceed with surgery.
- Consider POP-guided lithotripsy for pancreatic duct stones 5 mm or greater, stones recalcitrant to standard endoscopic retrograde pancreatography methods, and/or stones associated with downstream stricture for concurrent POP-guided stricturoplasty.
- Consider POP to rule out occult main-duct IPMN in patients with previously presumed idiopathic chronic pancreatitis and pancreatic duct dilatation.
- Consider POP for removal of foreign bodies from the pancreatic duct, particularly if there is an associated downstream stricture for concurrent POP-guided stricturoplasty.

DISCLOSURE

Y. Hanada—None. R.J. Shah—Consultant for Boston Scientific, Olympus, and Dragonfly.

SUPPLEMENTARY DATA

Supplementary data to this article can be found online at https://doi.org/10.1016/j.giec.2024.02.007.

REFERENCES

1. Shah RJ. Innovations in Intraductal Endoscopy: Cholangioscopy and Pancreatoscopy. Gastrointest Endosc Clin N Am 2015;25(4):779–92.
2. Komanduri S, Thosani N, Abu Dayyeh BK, et al. Cholangiopancreatoscopy. Gastrointest Endosc 2016;84(2):209–21. https://doi.org/10.1016/j.gie.2016.03.013.
3. El H II, Brauer BC, Wani S, et al. Role of per-oral pancreatoscopy in the evaluation of suspected pancreatic duct neoplasia: a 13-year U.S. single-center experience. Gastrointest Endosc 2017;85(4):737–45.
4. Ringold DA, Shah RJ. Peroral pancreatoscopy in the diagnosis and management of intraductal papillary mucinous neoplasia and indeterminate pancreatic duct pathology. Gastrointest Endosc Clin N Am 2009;19(4):601–13.
5. van der Wiel SE, Stassen PMC, Poley JW, et al. Pancreatoscopy-guided electrohydraulic lithotripsy for the treatment of obstructive pancreatic duct stones: a prospective consecutive case series. Gastrointest Endosc 2022;95(5):905–14.e2.
6. Han S, Shah RJ. Cholangiopancreatoscopy-guided laser dissection and ablation for pancreas and biliary strictures and neoplasia. Endosc Int Open 2020;8(8):E1091–6.
7. Mittal C, Shah RJ. Pancreatoscopy-guided laser dissection and ablation for treatment of benign and neoplastic pancreatic disorders: an initial report (with videos). Gastrointest Endosc 2019;89(2):384–9.
8. Al-Shahrani AA, Swei E, Wani S, et al. Pancreatoscopy-guided retrieval of a migrated pancreatic duct stent. VideoGIE 2022;7(11):417–8.
9. SpyGlass DS II Direct Visualization System ebrochure. Available at: https://www.bostonscientific.com/content/dam/bostonscientific/endo/portfolio-group/SpyGlass%20DS/SpyGlass-DS-System-ebrochure.pdf. [Accessed 1 September 2023].
10. Arnelo U, Siiki A, Swahn F, et al. Single-operator pancreatoscopy is helpful in the evaluation of suspected intraductal papillary mucinous neoplasms (IPMN). Pancreatology 2014;14(6):510–4.
11. Fritz S, Klauss M, Bergmann F, et al. Pancreatic main-duct involvement in branch-duct IPMNs: an underestimated risk. Ann Surg. Nov 2014;260(5):848–55, discussion 855-6.
12. Iqbal S, Stevens PD. Cholangiopancreatoscopy for targeted biopsies of the bile and pancreatic ducts. Gastrointest Endosc Clin N Am 2009;19(4):567–77.
13. Arnelo U, Valente R, Scandavini CM, et al. Intraoperative pancreatoscopy can improve the detection of skip lesions during surgery for intraductal papillary mucinous neoplasia: A pilot study. Pancreatology 2023. https://doi.org/10.1016/j.pan.2023.06.006.
14. Sauvanet A, Couvelard A, Belghiti J. Role of frozen section assessment for intraductal papillary and mucinous tumor of the pancreas. World J Gastrointest Surg 2010;2(10):352–8.

15. Han S, Raijman I, Machicado JD, et al. Per Oral Pancreatoscopy Identification of Main-duct Intraductal Papillary Mucinous Neoplasms and Concomitant Pancreatic Duct Stones: Not Mutually Exclusive. Pancreas 2019;48(6):792–4.
16. Brauer BC, Fukami N, Chen YK. Direct cholangioscopy with narrow-band imaging, chromoendoscopy, and argon plasma coagulation of intraductal papillary mucinous neoplasm of the bile duct (with videos). Gastrointest Endosc 2008; 67(3):574–6.
17. Brown NG, Camilo J, McCarter M, et al. Refractory Jaundice From Intraductal Papillary Mucinous Neoplasm Treated With Cholangioscopy-Guided Radiofrequency Ablation. ACG Case Rep J 2016;3(3):202–4.
18. Hara T, Yamaguchi T, Ishihara T, et al. Diagnosis and patient management of intraductal papillary-mucinous tumor of the pancreas by using peroral pancreatoscopy and intraductal ultrasonography. Gastroenterology 2002;122(1):34–43.
19. Itoi T, Sofuni A, Itokawa F, et al. Initial experience of peroral pancreatoscopy combined with narrow-band imaging in the diagnosis of intraductal papillary mucinous neoplasms of the pancreas (with videos). Gastrointest Endosc 2007; 66(4):793–7.
20. Kishimoto Y, Okano N, Ito K, et al. Peroral Pancreatoscopy with Videoscopy and Narrow-Band Imaging in Intraductal Papillary Mucinous Neoplasms with Dilatation of the Main Pancreatic Duct. Clin Endosc 2022;55(2):270–8.
21. Mounzer R, Austin GL, Wani S, et al. Per-oral video cholangiopancreatoscopy with narrow-band imaging for the evaluation of indeterminate pancreaticobiliary disease. Gastrointest Endosc 2017;85(3):509–17.
22. Ogura T, Hirose Y, Ueno S, et al. Prospective registration study of diagnostic yield and sample size in forceps biopsy using a novel device under digital cholangioscopy guidance with macroscopic on-site evaluation. J Hepatobiliary Pancreat Sci 2023;30(5):686–92.
23. Ammann RW, Muench R, Otto R, et al. Evolution and regression of pancreatic calcification in chronic pancreatitis. A prospective long-term study of 107 patients. Gastroenterology 1988;95(4):1018–28.
24. Kitano M, Gress TM, Garg PK, et al. International consensus guidelines on interventional endoscopy in chronic pancreatitis. Recommendations from the working group for the international consensus guidelines for chronic pancreatitis in collaboration with the International Association of Pancreatology, the American Pancreatic Association, the Japan Pancreas Society, and European Pancreatic Club. Pancreatology 2020;20(6):1045–55.
25. Bachmann K, Tomkoetter L, Kutup A, et al. Is the Whipple procedure harmful for long-term outcome in treatment of chronic pancreatitis? 15-years follow-up comparing the outcome after pylorus-preserving pancreatoduodenectomy and Frey procedure in chronic pancreatitis. Ann Surg 2013;258(5):815–20, discussion 820-1.
26. Hutchins RR, Hart RS, Pacifico M, et al. Long-term results of distal pancreatectomy for chronic pancreatitis in 90 patients. Ann Surg 2002;236(5):612–8.
27. Sakorafas GH, Farnell MB, Farley DR, et al. Long-term results after surgery for chronic pancreatitis. Int J Pancreatol 2000;27(2):131–42.
28. Contreras-Ramírez JRD, Luis C, et al. Puestow procedure: results in 19 years of institutional experience. Cir Gen 2021;43(1):15–22.
29. Han S, Miley A, Akshintala V, et al. Per-oral pancreatoscopy-guided lithotripsy vs. extracorporeal shock wave lithotripsy for treating refractory main pancreatic duct stones in chronic pancreatitis: Protocol for an open-label multi-center randomized clinical trial. Pancreatology 2022;22(8):1120–5.

30. van Huijgevoort NCM, Veld JV, Fockens P, et al. Success of extracorporeal shock wave lithotripsy and ERCP in symptomatic pancreatic duct stones: a systematic review and meta-analysis. Endosc Int Open 2020;8(8):E1070–85.
31. Dumonceau JM, Costamagna G, Tringali A, et al. Treatment for painful calcified chronic pancreatitis: extracorporeal shock wave lithotripsy versus endoscopic treatment: a randomised controlled trial. Gut 2007;56(4):545–52.
32. Strand DS, Law RJ, Yang D, et al. AGA Clinical Practice Update on the Endoscopic Approach to Recurrent Acute and Chronic Pancreatitis: Expert Review. Gastroenterology 2022;163(4):1107–14.
33. Han S, Shah RJ. ERCP with Digital Pancreatoscopy-Guided Stone Fragmentation: Breaking Up Is Easy to Do. Dig Dis Sci 2019;64(5):1059–61.
34. De Luca L, Repici A, Koçollari A, et al. Pancreatoscopy: An update. World J Gastrointest Endosc 2019;11(1):22–30.
35. McCarty TR, Sobani Z, Rustagi T. Per-oral pancreatoscopy with intraductal lithotripsy for difficult pancreatic duct stones: a systematic review and meta-analysis. Endosc Int Open 2020;8(10):E1460–70.
36. Ogura T, Okuda A, Imanishi M, et al. Electrohydraulic Lithotripsy for Pancreatic Duct Stones Under Digital Single-Operator Pancreatoscopy (with Video). Dig Dis Sci 2019;64(5):1377–82.
37. Miyabe K, Yoshida M, Hayashi K. Pancreatic stone extraction using a pancreatoscopy-directed, thin-sheathed basket catheter. Dig Endosc 2023; 35(1):e1–2.
38. Attwell AR, Patel S, Kahaleh M, et al. ERCP with per-oral pancreatoscopy-guided laser lithotripsy for calcific chronic pancreatitis: a multicenter U.S. experience. Gastrointest Endosc 2015;82(2):311–8.
39. Aldoukhi AH, Roberts WW, Hall TL, et al. Holmium Laser Lithotripsy in the New Stone Age: Dust or Bust? Front Surg 2017;4:57.
40. Jonica ER, Shah RJ. Pancreatoscopy-guided laser dissection of obstructing pancreatic duct stricture: pancreas-preserving endotherapy. VideoGIE 2022; 7(4):146–8.
41. Leonor PA, Miley A, Al-Shahrani A, et al. Endoscopic treatment of a refractory benign biliary stricture using cholangioscopy-guided thulium laser stricturoplasty. VideoGIE 2022;7(7):256–8.
42. Johanson JF, Schmalz MJ, Geenen JE. Incidence and risk factors for biliary and pancreatic stent migration. Gastrointest Endosc May-Jun 1992;38(3):341–6.
43. Price LH, Brandabur JJ, Kozarek RA, et al. Good stents gone bad: endoscopic treatment of proximally migrated pancreatic duct stents. Gastrointest Endosc 2009;70(1):174–9.
44. Kawaguchi Y, Lin JC, Kawashima Y, et al. Risk factors for migration, fracture, and dislocation of pancreatic stents. Gastroenterol Res Pract 2015;2015:365457.
45. Asif S, Kalpala R, Reddy DN. Peroral pancreatoscopy-assisted removal of internally migrated fractured pancreatic stent. Endoscopy 2020;52(10):E359.
46. Shah RJ, Langer DA, Antillon MR, et al. Cholangioscopy and cholangioscopic forceps biopsy in patients with indeterminate pancreaticobiliary pathology. Clin Gastroenterol Hepatol 2006;4(2):219–25.
47. de Jong DM, Stassen PMC, Groot Koerkamp B, et al. The role of pancreatoscopy in the diagnostic work-up of intraductal papillary mucinous neoplasms: a systematic review and meta-analysis. Endoscopy 2023;55(1):25–35.
48. Trindade AJ, Benias PC, Kurupathi P, et al. Digital pancreatoscopy in the evaluation of main duct intraductal papillary mucinous neoplasm: a multicenter study. Endoscopy 2018;50(11):1095–8.

49. Crippa S, Partelli S, Falconi M. Extent of surgical resections for intraductal papillary mucinous neoplasms. World J Gastrointest Surg 2010;2(10):347–51.
50. Roggin KK, Rudloff U, Blumgart LH, et al. Central pancreatectomy revisited. J Gastrointest Surg 2006;10(6):804–12.
51. Tyberg A, Raijman I, Siddiqui A, et al. Digital Pancreaticocholangioscopy for Mapping of Pancreaticobiliary Neoplasia: Can We Alter the Surgical Resection Margin? J Clin Gastroenterol 2019;53(1):71–5.
52. Attwell AR, Brauer BC, Chen YK, et al. Endoscopic retrograde cholangiopancreatography with per oral pancreatoscopy for calcific chronic pancreatitis using endoscope and catheter-based pancreatoscopes: a 10-year single-center experience. Pancreas 2014;43(2):268–74.
53. Brewer Gutierrez OI, Raijman I, Shah RJ, et al. Safety and efficacy of digital single-operator pancreatoscopy for obstructing pancreatic ductal stones. Endosc Int Open 2019;7(7):E896–903.
54. Guzmán-Calderón E, Martinez-Moreno B, Casellas JA, et al. Per-oral pancreatoscopy-guided lithotripsy for the endoscopic management of pancreatolithiasis: A systematic review and meta-analysis. J Dig Dis 2021;22(10):572–81.
55. de Rijk FEM, Stassen PMC, van der Wiel SE, et al. Long-term outcomes of pancreatoscopy-guided electrohydraulic lithotripsy for the treatment of obstructive pancreatic duct stones. Endosc Int Open 2023;11(03):E296–304.
56. Veld JV, van Huijgevoort NCM, Boermeester MA, et al. A systematic review of advanced endoscopy-assisted lithotripsy for retained biliary tract stones: laser, electrohydraulic or extracorporeal shock wave. Endoscopy 2018;50(9):896–909.

Endoscopic Management of Pain due to Chronic Pancreatitis

Arjun Kundra, MD[a], Daniel S. Strand, MD[b],
Vanessa M. Shami, MD[c],*

KEYWORDS

- Chronic pancreatitis • Pancreatic duct stones • Pancreatic duct obstruction
- Extracorporeal shockwave lithotripsy • ESWL • Celiac plexus block • Pain

KEY POINTS

- Pain secondary to chronic pancreatitis is a poorly understood and complex phenomenon.
- Treatments such as pancreatic duct decompression secondary to strictures, stones, or inflammatory and neoplastic processes are the mainstay of endoscopic therapy.
- For continued pain despite endoscopic treatment, endoscopic ultrasound -guided celiac block may be entertained; however, data are not robust on its effectiveness.

THE CLINICAL PROBLEM OF PAIN IN CHRONIC PANCREATITIS

Abdominal pain secondary to chronic pancreatitis (CP) is a vexing problem that results in a significant decrease in quality of life (QOL)[1] for patients and high costs to health care systems.[2] Classically, pain of pancreatic origin is described as episodic and localized to the mid-epigastrium with radiation to the back. While this description of pain is highly consistent in patients with acute pancreatitis, it does not conform particularly well to the variable presentations of pain in patients with CP.[3,4]

Historically, pain in CP was siloed into 2 discrete patterns (Type A and Type B) based upon the natural history observed in the cohort study by *Ammann and colleagues.*[5] Type A pain was described as *episodic* in nature, typically less than 2 weeks in duration, with symptom-free intervals between each episode. Type B pain, on the other hand, was defined by *persistent and daily pain*, which could also be accompanied by exacerbation(s). The North American Pancreatitis II (NAPS2) study group later demonstrated that those individuals with *persistent pain (Type B)* were also more likely

[a] Department of Gastroenterology and Hepatology, University of Virginia, Charlottesville, VA, USA; [b] Department of Gastroenterology, University of Virginia, Charlottesville, VA, USA; [c] Department of Medicine, University of Virginia, Charlottesville, VA, USA
* Corresponding author. Digestive Health Center, University of Virginia Health, Box 800701, Charlottesville, VA 22908.
E-mail address: vms4e@uvahealth.org

Gastrointest Endoscopy Clin N Am 34 (2024) 433–448
https://doi.org/10.1016/j.giec.2024.02.003
1052-5157/24/© 2024 Elsevier Inc. All rights reserved.
giendo.theclinics.com

to experience adverse health outcomes such as reduced QOL, disability, repetitive hospital admissions, and/or long-term opioid-use.[6] Complicating matters, pain is not ubiquitous in CP, as previously believed. Some patients, for reasons that are not entirely transparent, have absolutely no symptoms despite a radiographic diagnosis of CP.[7] This broad variability in clinical presentation underscores the complex milieu of pain in CP.[2]

Current expert consensus regarding pain in CP holds that it is extremely unreliable to objectively assess by the degree of end-organ pathology alone.[2,8] Pain is fundamentally a complex experience, characterized by sensory input subject to interpretation through myriad individualized factors.[2,6,9] Indeed, the subset of patients who experience severe pain due to altered nociception in CP may be uniquely susceptible in ways that were unappreciated in the past.[9] For example, a recent observational study suggests that patients with persistent pain from CP have a distinctly different profile of circulating chemokines and cytokines than those who do not.[10] Additionally, testing of patients from the NAPS2 cohort demonstrates a clear association of genetic loci for major depression in the fraction of patients who experience constant-severe pain from CP.[9,11] Novel differences such as these serve to underscore the complex interplay of central nervous system pathways, genetic predisposition, and biochemical and psychological cofactors that contribute to pain in patients with CP. None of these are intuitively accessible to the practicing endoscopist as a target for pancreatic endotherapy. This understanding is the basis for the growing notion that reflexive endoscopy for pain in CP is no longer broadly recommended but should be considered thoughtfully in the context of each patient with CP.[12]

Local mechanisms can also influence the development of pain in CP, and these factors are often felt to be more amenable to direct intervention.[13] Examples of these may include the development of local inflammation due to a discernible duct injury (ie, a duct leak), pancreatic ductal hypertension due to stricture and/or calculus, or the development of obstruction due to an inflammatory mass (eg, groove or para duodenal pancreatitis). Prior articles have addressed, in detail, the evidence regarding managing many of these specific structural complications of pancreatitis. Pain, which is refractory to conservative measures, is the most common reason why patients with CP are hospitalized, or are referred for surgery or endoscopic intervention.[2]

Endoscopic therapy for CP has mainly focused on decompression of pancreatic duct (PD) obstruction and splanchnic neural blockade targeting ganglia that innervate abdominal organs such as the pancreas. This section focuses on endoscopic pain management in patients with CP.

PANCREATIC DUCT OBSTRUCTION

Of the reasons for intervention typically cited by the endoscopist, pain due to pancreatic ductal hypertension is by far the most common.[14] Pancreatic duct obstruction can occur due to the progressive formation of calculi, often in the setting of fibroinflammatory strictures within the outflow tract of pancreatic secretion. Pain in this setting has been frequently attributed to increased pancreatic duct and parenchymal pressure or, possibly, local oxidative stress and ischemia. Pain due to PD obstruction is frequently characterized as *colicky* in nature and often *post-prandial*.[2,11] Despite the PD hypertension hypothesis, the results of studies designed to assess the correlation between PD pressure and symptoms have been mixed. Not all patients with elevated pancreatic duct pressures experience pain, and objectively measurable reductions in duct pressures do not reliably improve symptoms.[15,16]

Despite the lack of support for the "pressure" etiopathology, there is evidence from the NAPS2 cohort (and elsewhere) that patients with abdominal pain do benefit from endoscopic intervention in CP.[17] Response rates to pancreatic intervention, typically endoscopic placement of a pancreatic stent in retrospective cohorts are highly variable and depend considerably upon context and design. Results range from no statistical benefit to significant relief of pain in 85% of included patients.[17–19] Nearly all of the existing data are derived from observational, retrospective, and heterogeneous studies. As such, our understanding of the expected results of pancreatic endotherapy is subject to considerable bias and thus should be interpreted cautiously. Controlled, randomized data are rare, and where studies do exist, they are far from definitive.[20]

Patient selection is also essential when offering endoscopic therapy to those with CP, and the presence of complicating variables (such as ongoing alcohol and cigarette use) makes any accurate prediction of benefit extremely challenging.[13] Perhaps in recognition of the overall lack of high-quality data in this milieu, general guidance regarding the role of endoscopic intervention in CP is available from multiple societies.[12–14] Specific intervention(s) performed by gastrointestinal endoscopists may include endoscopic retrograde pancreatography (ERCP)-directed relief of obstruction, remodeling of PD stricture(s), and elimination of stones. Endoscopic ultrasound (EUS) is typically employed to deliver splanchnic nociceptive blockade via the celiac plexus or ganglion.[12,14]

Preprocedural Planning

Before undertaking any endoscopic therapy, cross-sectional imaging is paramount to determine ductal diameter, level of obstruction, presence, size, and number of calculi and concomitant strictures, presence of parenchymal atrophy or extensive parenchymal calcifications, and findings suggestive of an underlying malignancy. Computed tomography (CT) and MRI are complementary. MRI with secretin stimulation provides the best assessment of the PD and is preferable in the setting of a disconnected main PD.

PANCREATIC SPHINCTEROTOMY

PD orifice sphincterotomy is a commonly performed endoscopic intervention. It is typically done with the intent to relieve papillary sphincter stenosis or allow for improved duct access for endoscopic instruments. PD sphincterotomy can also facilitate passage of pancreatoscopes (10Fr caliber) and luminal delivery of main duct calculi (before or after fragmentation) (**Fig. 1**). Typically, PD sphincterotomy is an adjuvant maneuver, though this can be a primary therapy when sphincter sclerosis is felt to be the driver of patient symptoms in the absence of upstream ductal obstruction in the setting of chronic pancreatitis.[14] In patients with pancreas divisum, minor papilla sphincterotomy may be considered to reduce episodic attacks of acute pancreatitis or to provide pain relief.[12] It should be noted that patients who develop pancreatitis in the setting of divisum rarely do so in isolation. Nearly half of such patients will have an identifiable secondary cause, such as a cystic fibrosis transmembrane conductance regulator mutation, which can make it challenging to determine if endoscopic therapy will be beneficial.[21]

PANCREATIC DUCT STENTING

Main pancreatic duct (MPD) stent placement is one of the most performed endoscopic procedures to affect pancreatic duct decompression (**Fig. 2**). Some endoscopists place a main pancreatic stent across any obstruction to assess pain relief before

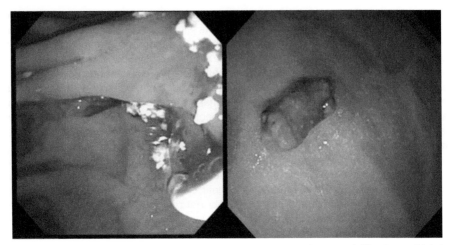

Fig. 1. Pancreatic duct (PD) calculi. The white appearance is due to calcification, which is common with PDstones.

embarking on attempts to definitively resolve ductal pathology, which often requires multiple, sometimes labor-intensive (eg, Pancreatoscopy with intraductal lithotripsy) endoscopic procedures.

While there is little doubt that endoscopic ductal therapy with balloon dilation and placement of 1 or more stents can mitigate the radiographic appearance of a

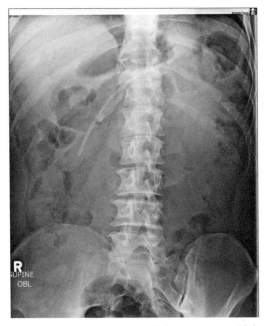

Fig. 2. Long plastic PD stent placed into the tail of the pancreas, with large, calcific pancreatic duct stone visible at the level of the pancreatic neck.

pancreatic duct stricture, the efficacy of this intervention for pain remains subject to considerable debate.[12] As stated previously, the causal relationship between pancreatic ductal hypertension and pain is unclear,[15] as is the fundamental expectation that relief of pressure will ameliorate pain.[16]

The largest retrospective, multicenter cohort study included over 1000 patients with CP who underwent MPD stent placement for a dominant main pancreatic duct stricture. Of these, 57% of the patients demonstrated significant pain relief at long-term follow-up (mean of 4.9 years). An additional 19% of those included had significant symptom improvement but also required ongoing endoscopic intervention.[22] Modern cohort studies, which provide the same level of evidence for pain relief, typically demonstrate similar findings. One such experience, by *Tringali and colleagues*, reported durable pain relief in 75% of the treated patients following stent removal for up to approximately 180 months after stricture remediation.[23]

Current multi-society (Internation Association of Pancreatology [IAP]/American Pancreatic Association [APA]/Japan Pancreas Society [JPS]/European Pancreas Club [EPC]) guidance argues that up to 60% of appropriate patients who are selected for MPD stent placement can expect to experience both short-term (<2 years) and long-term (>5 years) symptom relief.[24] These authors acknowledge that the data upon which this recommendation is based are heterogeneous, low quality (by GRADE methodology), and prototypically observational.

Despite these limitations, it was recommended by Drewes and colleagues to target patients early in their disease course and to consider prioritizing patients with a single dominant stricture or stone in the pancreatic head. Data from NAPS2 also support this recommendation, as patients with a shorter disease duration appear more likely to respond to endoscopic therapy (4 vs 40 months; $P = .017$).[17] Despite observational data, durable relief of symptoms remains a significant problem,[20] particularly because the natural history of pain in chronic pancreatitis appears independent of disease duration[3] for reasons discussed in the preamble. While endoscopic decompression is unquestionably useful, in the authors' estimation, the perfect positioning of ERCP-directed stent placement in patients with CP is not well defined. The decision to proceed with ERCP, especially when the endpoint is pain relief, should be thoughtfully considered and transparently discussed with prospective patients.

When endoscopic intervention is selected, plastic PD stents are typically placed to bridge a stricture in the MPD. This can be done as singular therapy or following endoscopic balloon dilation to a diameter appropriate for the caliber of the upstream pancreatic duct. These plastic stents are typically exchanged at 3-month intervals but may be left for a longer duration if larger (ie, 10 French) in caliber.[14] Overall treatment duration typically exceeds 12 months, as shorter treatment periods are associated with inferior outcomes.[14,19] The preferred strategy is to place and, on exchanges, either upsize or add multiple plastic stents in parallel to allow for improved caliber of the strictured ductal segment during remodeling.[12]

To reduce the number of ERCP procedures required to achieve durable stricture resolution, fully covered self-expanding metal stents (fcSEMS) have been used for this indication. Several individual studies[25] and a recent systemic review and meta-analysis[26] have examined this practice. Both plastic stents and FcSEMS are generally observed to resolve MPD strictures in most patients (approximately 90%) and are associated with similar rates of pain relief (88% vs 89%).[26] Importantly, however, significantly more AEs were observed in patients who underwent treatment with fcSEMS compared to plastic stents (39% vs 14%).[26] Due to the preferable safety profile, this expert group of authors favors upsizing or placing coaxial parallel plastic stents to treat MPD strictures. This practice is in keeping with recommendations proffered in the American Gastroenterology Association Clinical Practice Update by *Strand and colleagues.*[12]

It should also be noted that MPD stent placement is not an entirely benign affair, and AEs have been reported in up to 10% to 20% of patients. Most commonly, this is due to stent migration or the development of a stricture at the proximal (upstream) end of an indwelling stent.[17] Given these observations, the authors' typical practice favors the placement of longer MPD stents that terminate in the tail of the pancreas. This decision is largely agnostic of the location of the stricture to be treated (head or body), but rather to avoid AEs, as the authors' anecdotal experience suggests that stents that terminate at the site of directional transition (ie, the genu) within the PD are the most problematic.

PANCREATIC DUCT STONE MANAGEMENT

Pancreatic duct calculi can be a significant challenge to manage, as they are a different composition than biliary stones. Specifically, PD stones are often composed of a small inner nidus of sulfur and chlorine with successive outer shell layers of calcium carbonate.[27] This chemical composition results in a high-density, rigid stone that can prove refractory to standard ERCP maneuvers. Additionally, they typically form *in situ* and may result in cast-like duct obstruction that can impede the progress of (or break) endoscopic instruments such as dilation and extraction balloons.[28] Obstructing stones that are small (<4-5 mm) and located within the head and neck of the PD are the most amenable to endoscopic therapy.[12] Larger stones (>5 mm) may require lithotripsy, which can be performed via ERCP-directed techniques or extracorporeal shock wave lithotripsy (ESWL).[29] It should also be noted that the presence of a stone is not a *sine qua non* for intervention. Many patients possess *extensive* calcific chronic pancreatitis in the absence of clinical symptoms, including pain.[7] In this setting, preventing future complications (such as the development of diabetes) is often cited as the rationale for treating asymptomatic stones, though data supporting such practice remain limited.[30] Once the decision is made to pursue intervention for a PD stone, management is often predicated on the location and size of the target.

Management of small stones (<4 mm) can usually be accomplished by conventional ERCP techniques. In most cases, fluoroscopically directed extraction using a standard retrieval balloon or basket after endoscopic pancreatic sphincterotomy will suffice. Sometimes, balloon dilation of the papillary orifice or a focal stricture downstream to the stone may be necessary as an adjunct maneuver.[31] If a stone cannot be removed in a single session, endoscopic stent across the obstruction is typically performed.[32]

Larger (> 5 mm) or impacted stones often require ESWL (**Figs. 3–5**). ESWL is the oldest and perhaps most widely studied intervention for refractory PD calculi. Although the availability of ESWL in the United States is limited, it remains a highly effective intervention for fragmentation of PD stones.[14,29] This can be performed alone or in combination with subsequent ERCPs to retrieve fragments. A randomized controlled trial of 55 patients by *Dumonceau and colleagues* suggested that ESWL alone may be comparable to a combination of ESWL and ERCP to relieve pancreatitis-related pain.[29] Additional observational studies[33] also favor ESWL as an effective sole intervention for pain. Accordingly, multiple guidelines include ESWL as an important modality in the schema for PD stone management.[14,24] Relying entirely on ESWL, however, can be problematic. A Japanese study by *Tadenuma and colleagues* observed that in patients who have incomplete stone removal at the time of

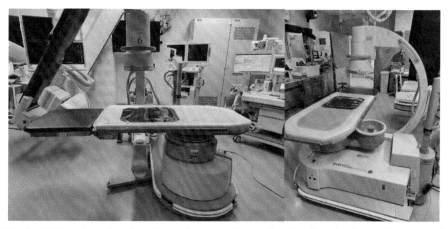

Fig. 3. ESWL setup, showing C-arm for targeting and delivering shocks, to be targeted within the field of the waterbed section.

initial therapy, symptoms of abdominal pain following ESWL relapse much more commonly.[34] Thus, complete clearance of stones from the pancreatic duct by ERCP should be considered in patients who have residual stones following ESWL.[14] The ideal method and timeline to ensure spontaneous passage of pancreatic duct residua prior to embarking on a subsequent ERCP is not well established.[34]

ERCP with single-operator pancreatoscopy-directed lithotripsy is an alternative to ESWL. Specific treatment modalities delivered by this method include electrohydraulic lithotripsy (EHL) and laser lithotripsy (LL). Intraductal therapy is subject to significant endoscopist enthusiasm, given the limited availability of ESWL in the United States and the prospect of PD clearance in a "single session." Retrospective data on these techniques, typically performed at expert tertiary care centers reveal a high degree of technical success comparable to ESWL.[28,33,35–37] These data further support the notion that pancreatoscopy-directed lithotripsy is safe and likely effective, though it is often technically challenging, and thus, generalizability beyond expert centers may be limited. It should also be noted that some retrospective studies of intraductal therapy combine patients treated with EHL and LL into a single cohort

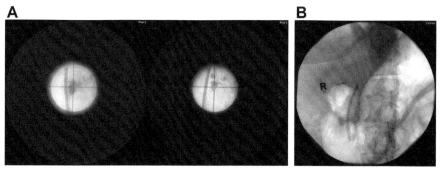

Fig. 4. (*A*) Stone targeting and progression of PD stone fracturing with extracorporeal shock wave lithotripsy shock deliverance in a patient. (*B*) Complete clearance of obstructing PD stone in the same patient.

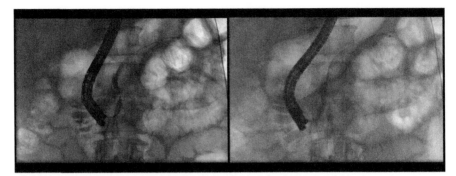

Fig. 5. Resolution of pancreatic duct patency with clearance of large pancreatic duct stone at the level of the neck of the pancreas.

despite these treatments having different operating variables.[38] Additionally, the cost burden of intraductal treatment compared to ESWL is not well established, though it may favor the former. At present, there are no high-quality, randomized data that provide the means to make a definitive choice between these 2 modalities for PD stone destruction—though this may be forthcoming.[39]

CELIAC PLEXUS BLOCK

The celiac plexus is a network of 1 to 5 ganglia that relays preganglionic sympathetic and parasympathetic efferent fibers and visceral sensory afferent fibers to the upper abdominal viscera, including the pancreas. It is in the vicinity of the celiac artery at its takeoff from the aorta. The celiac plexus can be identified by endoscopic ultrasound. First, the aorta is identified in the thorax and followed distally to its first major branch below the diaphragm, the celiac artery. The ganglia surround the celiac artery take-off and can often be individually visualized (**Fig. 6**).

CELIAC PLEXUS BLOCK/TECHNIQUE

In patients with CP, celiac plexus block (CPB) has been utilized to decrease pain with hopes of improving QOL and reducing narcotic use. The typical technique involves

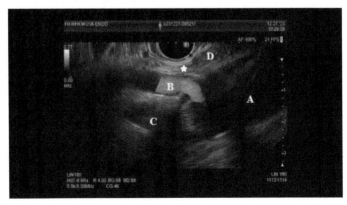

Fig. 6. Endosonographic image taken with a linear echoendoscope demonstrating the aorta (A), celiac artery takeoff, (B), superior mesenteric artery takeoff (C), diaphragm (D) and expected location for the celiac ganglion to target for injection (*star*), highlighted with eFlow.

injecting bupivacaine and triamcinolone into the celiac axis.[13] Contraindications include patients with esophageal strictures, altered anatomy precluding access to the proximal stomach, coagulopathy, or thrombocytopenia (platelet count <50,000/mm³).

Patients are given intravenous volume expansion (Lactated Ringer's or normal saline) before and during the procedure to minimize hypotension due to dilation of the splanchnic vasculature as a result of the block. Once the patient is sedated, the celiac axis is identified. The needle is inserted into the region of the celiac axis; aspiration is performed for several seconds to ensure that it is not in a vascular structure. A combination of 20 mL of 0.25% bupivacaine and 80 mg triamcinolone is injected into the plexus adjacent to the celiac artery takeoff. After completion of the procedure, patients are observed for hypotension for at least 1 hour.

Unilateral Versus Bilateral Injection

Since the plexus surrounds the celiac artery, instead of injecting the bupivacaine and triamcinolone on 1 side of the takeoff, known as the unilateral approach, some advocate for injection of half of the injectant on both sides of the celiac artery (bilateral approach). No robust data favor either the unilateral or bilateral approach. When reviewing the sparse data for CPB, in a prospective trial of 160 patients, bilateral CPB was found to be more effective.[40] Pain relief was 70.4% on day 7 in bilateral versus 45.9% in unilateral arm. However, another prospective randomized trial showed no difference in duration or time to onset of pain relief.[41]

Indirect Versus Direct Injection

Direct targeting of the ganglia has also been reported. However, the data are sparse. In a study, celiac plexus block (CPB) and celiac plexus neurolysis (CPN) were performed for CP and pancreatic cancer. For CP, four-fifth (80%) who received alcohol injection reported pain relief versus five-thirteenth (38%) receiving corticosteroid injection.[42] In a recent prospective study of patients with unresectable pancreatic cancer, those who underwent celiac ganglion neurolysis (CGN) had reduced survival time without improving pain, QOL, or AEs versus CPN. The patients who experienced increased post-procedural pain appeared to have improved results.[43] Whether these results are generalizable to patients with CP undergoing CPB is unclear.

CELIAC PLEXUS BLOCK/DATA

Several retrospective and prospective studies have demonstrated the technical success of EUS-CPB is as high as 95%.[40,41,44–48] However, its efficacy in pain relief is suboptimal, and 2 meta-analyses demonstrate disappointing response rates.[44,48] The first study, authored by *Kaufman and colleagues.*[44], included 6 trials with 221 patients who underwent EUS-CPB for CP. Pain relief was only reported in 51.46% of the patients included. The second meta-analysis, by *Puli and colleagues.*[48], included 9 studies with 376 patients. The response rate was higher, with 59% reporting symptom improvement; however, the degree of reported pain relief was modest, and most patients included in the analysis continued to require analgesic medications. Such meta-analyses are subject to considerable methodologic limitations, and these 2 examples notably included abstract-level data and no higher quality randomized trials.

CPB is even more disappointing when stringent criteria to define pain relief are applied. In a study by *Stevens and colleagues*, 40 patients with abdominal pain secondary to CP were randomized to receive CPB with either triamcinolone and bupivacaine or bupivacaine alone (control group).[49] Following CPB, the patients were assessed at 30 days with a primary endpoint defined as a decrease in the pain disability index of 10 or more. Although there was no difference between groups, the results of CPB were uniformly dismal: Only 14.3% of patients who received triamcinolone met the primary endpoint for pain relief versus 15.8% for controls.[49]

Conversely, a randomized trial by *Gress and colleagues*[47] compared EUS to CT-guided CPB for pain in patients with CP. In this study, approximately (5/10) 50% of the patients in the EUS group experienced significant short-term pain reduction. Continued benefit was noted in approximately 40% of the responders at 8 weeks and 30% at 24 weeks. The EUS-directed approach was superior to CT-CPB, where only one-fourth (25%) experienced a significant reduction in abdominal pain.[47] The same authors later published a prospective, single-center experience of EUS-CPB on 90 patients with CP.[47] In this series, 55% (50/90) of the patients reported significant short-term improvement in objective pain scores. This benefit appeared transient, however, as only 26% of the responders had a persistent benefit by 12 weeks, and 10% at 24 weeks.[47]

While data on the efficacy of EUS-CPB on pain relief in patients with CP are generally underwhelming, there are data to support the role of serial CPB in patients who demonstrate prior benefit.[13,45] Enthusiasm for this approach should be tempered, however, as the duration of response remains limited (approximately 10 weeks), and there is no apparent benefit associated with repeated injections for those who do not respond initially.

Current expert and societal recommendations regarding the utility of CPB in CP are variable and sometimes appear conflicting.[12,13] The observed discrepancy is principally due to differences in the interpretation of existing low-quality evidence filtered through the perceived risk of CPB against alternative treatments. The American College of gastroenterology (ACG) recommends "considering" celiac plexus block for CP-related pain,[13] whereas the recent AGA Clinical Practice Update counsels that "CPB should not be routinely performed" for this indication.[12] While seemingly at odds, when read closely, these recommendations are, in fact, very similar. The decision to proceed with CPB in selected patients with debilitating pain in whom other therapeutic measures have failed can be considered on a case-by-case basis, but only after discussion of the uncertain benefit of this intervention and its procedural risks.[12]

CELIAC PLEXUS BLOCK/ADVERSE EVENTS

AEs are observed in up to 40% of patients, including diarrhea and hypotension, which are the most common.[42,46,47,50] Diarrhea is related to the blockade of sympathetic innervation to the abdominal viscera and results from unopposed parasympathetic stimulation. Hypotension occurs due to the dilation of the splanchnic vasculature and can be treated with intravenous volume expansion.

Fortunately, significant AE from CPB are rare and occur in <1% of patients. Reported AEs include abscess formation, bleeding, and intravascular injection. Reports of paralysis, which are extremely rare, have been limited to alcohol-based celiac neurolysis.[45,51–55]

LIMITATIONS OF ENDOSCOPIC THERAPY AND THE CASE FOR SURGERY

Newer guidelines published in 2021 on the management of CP also suggest that long-term repeated endoscopic treatment beyond 2 to 3 years should not be used to treat pain in patients with chronic pancreatitis. However, the strength of this recommendation was weak.[56] This is likely due to the nature of the pain becoming more neuropathic as the course of the disease progresses. In cases where pain is exceptionally challenging to manage, surgery can be considered. Although the superiority of surgery in managing CPpain has been demonstrated in the Early Surgery versus optimal Current step-up prActice for chronic PancrEatitis (ESCAPE) randomized controlled trial,[20] endoscopic therapies are still considered first-line as they are less invasive and have low AE rates. Surgical treatment options include distal pancreatectomy, Whipple's operation to achieve partial resection, and Puestow procedure for improved drainage. Additionally, there are combined procedures such as Frey's, Berne, and Beger operations for resection and improved drainage.[57]

CLINICS CARE POINTS

- Identifying the characteristics of pancreatic pain, and structural causes such as stones or strictures is instrumental in deciding whether endoscopic therapy is indicated and which type of therapy would likely be most effective.

- Main pancreatic duct stent placement for management of pancreatic duct stictures in carefully selected patients can provide both short and long term pain relief in >50% of patients. Success is more likely if patients are targeted early in their disease course.

- Fully covered self-expanding metal stents carry a higher adverse event rate for main pancreatic duct strictures, and as such coaxial parallel plastic stents is favored.

- Extracorporeal shock wave lithotripsy (ESWL) is useful in management of larger pancreatic stones and additional ERCP for stone clearance after ESWL can be considered in patients who have residual stones following ERCP.

- Intraductal therapy for pancreatic duct stones with electohydraulic lithotripsy is a reasonable alternative to ESWL Pitfalls:.

- Offering endoscopic therapy for duct decompression without clear evidence of obstruction may result in unnecessary procedures and possible complications.

- The ideal method and timeline to ensure spontaneous passage of pancreatic duct residua after ESWL, prior to embarking on a subsequent ERCP is not well established.

SUMMARY

Pain from CP is multifactorial and not fully understood. Treatments such as pancreatic duct decompression secondary to strictures, stones, or inflammatory and neoplastic processes are the mainstay of endoscopic therapy. For continued pain despite endoscopic treatment, EUS-guided celiac block may be entertained; however, data are not robust on its effectiveness.

DISCLOSURE

A. Kundra and D.S. Strand has nothing to disclose. V.M. Shami: Consultant for Cook Medical, Olympus America, and Boston Scientific.

REFERENCES

1. Machicado JD, Amann ST, Anderson MA, et al. Quality of Life in Chronic Pancreatitis is Determined by Constant Pain, Disability/Unemployment, Current Smoking, and Associated Co-Morbidities. Am J Gastroenterol 2017;112:633–42. Available at: https://pubmed.ncbi.nlm.nih.gov/28244497/. [Accessed 27 December 2023].

2. Anderson MA, Akshintala V, Albers KM, et al. Mechanism, Assessment and Management of Pain in Chronic Pancreatitis: Recommendations of a Multidisciplinary Study Group. Pancreatology 2016;16:83. Available at: http://pmc/articles/PMC4761301/. [Accessed 27 December 2023].

3. Vipperla K, Kanakis A, Slivka A, et al. Natural course of pain in chronic pancreatitis is independent of disease duration. Pancreatology 2021;21:649–57. Available at: https://pubmed.ncbi.nlm.nih.gov/33674197/. [Accessed 27 December 2023].

4. Wilcox CM, Yadav D, Ye T, et al. Chronic pancreatitis pain pattern and severity are independent of abdominal imaging findings. Clin Gastroenterol Hepatol 2015;13: 552–60. Available at: https://pubmed.ncbi.nlm.nih.gov/25424572/. [Accessed 27 December 2023].

5. Ammann RW, Muellhaupt B, Akovbiantz A, et al. The natural history of pain in alcoholic chronic pancreatitis. Gastroenterology 1999;116:1132–40. Available at: https://pubmed.ncbi.nlm.nih.gov/10220505/. [Accessed 27 December 2023].

6. Mullady DK, Yadav D, Amann ST, et al. Type of pain, pain-associated complications, quality of life, disability and resource utilisation in chronic pancreatitis: a prospective cohort study. Gut 2011;60:77–84. Available at: https://pubmed.ncbi.nlm.nih.gov/21148579/. [Accessed 27 December 2023].

7. Ahmed A, Shah I, Bocchino R, et al. Natural history, clinical characteristics, outcomes, and long-term follow-up of pain-free chronic pancreatitis. Gastroenterol Rep (Oxf) 2023;11. Available at: https://pubmed.ncbi.nlm.nih.gov/37153703/. [Accessed 27 December 2023].

8. Pain HM. Pain terms: a list with definitions and notes on usage. Recommended by the IASP Subcommittee on Taxonomy. cir.nii.ac.jp. 1979 undefined. Available at: https://cir.nii.ac.jp/crid/1572543024166034688. [Accessed 27 December 2023].

9. Dunbar E, Greer PJ, Melhem N, et al. Constant-severe pain in chronic pancreatitis is associated with genetic loci for major depression in the NAPS2 cohort. J Gastroenterol 2020;55:1000–9. Available at: https://pubmed.ncbi.nlm.nih.gov/32681239/. [Accessed 27 December 2023].

10. Saloman JL, Tang G, Stello KM, et al. Serum biomarkers for chronic pancreatitis pain patterns. Pancreatology 2021;21:1411–8. Available at: https://pubmed.ncbi.nlm.nih.gov/34602367/. [Accessed 27 December 2023].

11. Dunbar EK, Saloman JL, Phillips AE, et al. Severe Pain in Chronic Pancreatitis Patients: Considering Mental Health and Associated Genetic Factors. J Pain Res 2021;14:773–84. Available at: https://pubmed.ncbi.nlm.nih.gov/33762844/. [Accessed 27 December 2023].

12. Strand DS, Law RJ, Yang D, et al. AGA clinical practice update on the endoscopic approach to recurrent acute and chronic pancreatitis: expert review. Gastroenterology; 2022. p. 163. Available at: https://pubmed.ncbi.nlm.nih.gov/36008176/. [Accessed 27 December 2023].

13. Gardner TB, Adler DG, Forsmark CE, et al. ACG clinical guideline: chronic pancreatitis. Am J Gastroenterol 2020;115:322–39. Available at: https://pubmed.ncbi.nlm.nih.gov/32022720/. [Accessed 27 December 2023].

14. Dumonceau JM, Delhaye M, Tringali A, et al. Endoscopic treatment of chronic pancreatitis: European Society of Gastrointestinal Endoscopy (ESGE) Guideline - Updated August 2018. Endoscopy 2019;51:179–93. Available at: https://pubmed.ncbi.nlm.nih.gov/30654394/. [Accessed 27 December 2023].

15. Novis BH, Bornman PC, Girdwood AW, et al. Endoscopic manometry of the pancreatic duct and sphincter zone in patients with chronic pancreatitis. Dig

Dis Sci 1985;30:225–8. Available at: https://pubmed.ncbi.nlm.nih.gov/3971834/. [Accessed 27 December 2023].

16. Renou C, Grandval P, Ville E, et al. Endoscopic treatment of the main pancreatic duct: correlations among morphology, manometry, and clinical follow-up. Int J Pancreatol 2000;27:143–9. Available at: https://pubmed.ncbi.nlm.nih.gov/10862513/. [Accessed 27 December 2023].

17. Clarke B, Slivka A, Tomizawa Y, et al. Endoscopic therapy is effective for patients with chronic pancreatitis. Clin Gastroenterol Hepatol 2012;10:795–802. Available at: https://pubmed.ncbi.nlm.nih.gov/22245964/. [Accessed 27 December 2023].

18. Seza K, Yamaguchi T, Ishihara T, et al. A long-term controlled trial of endoscopic pancreatic stenting for treatment of main pancreatic duct stricture in chronic pancreatitis. Hepato-Gastroenterology 2011;58:2128–31. Available at: https://pubmed.ncbi.nlm.nih.gov/22234084/. [Accessed 27 December 2023].

19. Eleftheriadis N, Dinu F, Delhaye M, et al. Long-term outcome after pancreatic stenting in severe chronic pancreatitis. Endoscopy 2005;37:223–30. Available at: https://pubmed.ncbi.nlm.nih.gov/18556820/. [Accessed 27 December 2023].

20. Issa Y, Kempeneers MA, Bruno MJ, et al. Effect of Early Surgery vs Endoscopy-First Approach on Pain in Patients With Chronic Pancreatitis: The ESCAPE Randomized Clinical Trial. JAMA 2020;323:237–47. Available at: https://pubmed.ncbi.nlm.nih.gov/31961419/. [Accessed 27 December 2023].

21. Bertin C, Pelletier AL, Vullierme MP, et al. Pancreas divisum is not a cause of pancreatitis by itself but acts as a partner of genetic mutations. Am J Gastroenterol 2012;107:311–7. Available at: https://pubmed.ncbi.nlm.nih.gov/22158025/. [Accessed 27 December 2023].

22. Rösch T, Daniel S, Scholz M, et al. Endoscopic treatment of chronic pancreatitis: a multicenter study of 1000 patients with long-term follow-up. Endoscopy 2002;34:765–71. Available at: https://pubmed.ncbi.nlm.nih.gov/12244496/. [Accessed 27 December 2023].

23. Tringali A, Bove V, Vadalà Di Prampero SF, et al. Long-term follow-up after multiple plastic stenting for refractory pancreatic duct strictures in chronic pancreatitis. Endoscopy 2019;51:930–5.

24. Drewes AM, Bouwense SAW, Campbell CM, et al. Guidelines for the understanding and management of pain in chronic pancreatitis. Pancreatology 2017;17:720–31. Available at: https://pubmed.ncbi.nlm.nih.gov/28734722/. [Accessed 27 December 2023].

25. Oh D, Lee JH, Song TJ, et al. Long-term outcomes of 6-mm diameter fully covered self-expandable metal stents in benign refractory pancreatic ductal stricture. Dig Endosc 2018;30:508–15. Available at: https://pubmed.ncbi.nlm.nih.gov/29453786/. [Accessed 27 December 2023].

26. Sofi AA, Khan MA, Ahmad S, et al. Comparison of clinical outcomes of multiple plastic stents and covered metal stent in refractory pancreatic ductal strictures in chronic pancreatitis- a systematic review and meta-analysis. Pancreatology 2021;21:854–61. Available at: https://pubmed.ncbi.nlm.nih.gov/33941467/. [Accessed 27 December 2023].

27. Jing ZP. Ultrastructure and elemental composition of pancreatic stones. Zhonghua Wai Ke Za Zhi 1990;28:421–3. Available at: https://europepmc.org/article/MED/2269050. [Accessed 27 December 2023].

28. Han S, Shah RJ, Brauer BC, et al. A Comparison of Endoscopic Retrograde Pancreatography With or Without Pancreatoscopy for Removal of Pancreatic Duct Stones. Pancreas 2019;48:690–7. Available at: https://pubmed.ncbi.nlm.nih.gov/31091217/. [Accessed 27 December 2023].

29. Dumonceau JM, Costamagna G, Tringali A, et al. Treatment for painful calcified chronic pancreatitis: extracorporeal shock wave lithotripsy versus endoscopic treatment: a randomised controlled trial. Gut 2007;56:545–52. Available at: https://pubmed.ncbi.nlm.nih.gov/17047101/. [Accessed 27 December 2023].

30. Talukdar R, Reddy DN, Tandan M, et al. Impact of ductal interventions on diabetes in patients with chronic pancreatitis. J Gastroenterol Hepatol 2021;36: 1226–34. Available at: https://pubmed.ncbi.nlm.nih.gov/33000865/. [Accessed 27 December 2023].

31. Bansal R, Patil G, Puri R, et al. Endoscopic pancreatic balloon sphincteroplasty for difficult to treat pancreatic stones and strictures: experience in 80 patients. Endosc Int Open 2017;5:E1229–34. Available at: https://pubmed.ncbi.nlm.nih. gov/29218314/. [Accessed 27 December 2023].

32. Choi EK, McHenry L, Watkins JL, et al. Use of intravenous secretin during extracorporeal shock wave lithotripsy to facilitate endoscopic clearance of pancreatic duct stones. Pancreatology 2012;12:272–5. Available at: https://pubmed.ncbi. nlm.nih.gov/22687384/. [Accessed 27 December 2023].

33. Vaysse T, Boytchev I, Antoni G, et al. Efficacy and safety of extracorporeal shock wave lithotripsy for chronic pancreatitis. Scand J Gastroenterol 2016;51:1380–5. Available at: https://pubmed.ncbi.nlm.nih.gov/27595309/. [Accessed 27 December 2023].

34. Tadenuma H, Ishihara T, Yamaguchi T, et al. Long-term results of extracorporeal shockwave lithotripsy and endoscopic therapy for pancreatic stones. Clin Gastroenterol Hepatol 2005;3:1128–35. Available at: https://pubmed.ncbi.nlm.nih.gov/ 16271345/. [Accessed 27 December 2023].

35. McCarty TR, Sobani Z, Rustagi T. Per-oral pancreatoscopy with intraductal lithotripsy for difficult pancreatic duct stones: a systematic review and meta-analysis. Endosc Int Open 2020;8:E1460–70. Available at: https://pubmed.ncbi.nlm.nih. gov/33043115/. [Accessed 27 December 2023].

36. Wiel SE, Stassen PMC, Poley JW, et al. Pancreatoscopy-guided electrohydraulic lithotripsy for the treatment of obstructive pancreatic duct stones: a prospective consecutive case series. Gastrointest Endosc 2022;95:905–14.e2. Available at: https://pubmed.ncbi.nlm.nih.gov/34906545/. [Accessed 27 December 2023].

37. Bekkali NLH, Murray S, Johnson GJ, et al. Pancreatoscopy-Directed Electrohydraulic Lithotripsy for Pancreatic Ductal Stones in Painful Chronic Pancreatitis Using SpyGlass. Pancreas 2017;46:528–30. Available at: https://pubmed.ncbi.nlm. nih.gov/28196019/. [Accessed 27 December 2023].

38. Brewer Gutierrez OI, Raijman I, Shah RJ, et al. Safety and efficacy of digital single-operator pancreatoscopy for obstructing pancreatic ductal stones. Endosc Int Open 2019;7:E896–903. Available at: https://pubmed.ncbi.nlm.nih.gov/ 31281875/. [Accessed 27 December 2023].

39. Olesen SS, Drewes AM, Gaud R, et al. Combined extracorporeal shock wave lithotripsy and endoscopic treatment for pain in chronic pancreatitis (SCHOKE trial): study protocol for a randomized, sham-controlled trial. Trials 2020;21. Available at: https://pubmed.ncbi.nlm.nih.gov/32299454/. [Accessed 27 December 2023].

40. Sahai AV, Lemelin V, Lam E, et al. Central vs. bilateral endoscopic ultrasound-guided celiac plexus block or neurolysis: a comparative study of short-term effectiveness. Am J Gastroenterol 2009;104:326–9. Available at: https://pubmed.ncbi. nlm.nih.gov/19174816/. [Accessed 27 December 2023].

41. LeBlanc JK, DeWitt J, Johnson C, et al. A prospective randomized trial of 1 versus 2 injections during EUS-guided celiac plexus block for chronic

pancreatitis pain. Gastrointest Endosc 2009;69:835–42. Available at: https://pubmed.ncbi.nlm.nih.gov/19136101/. [Accessed 27 December 2023].

42. Levy MJ, Topazian MD, Wiersema MJ, et al. Initial evaluation of the efficacy and safety of endoscopic ultrasound-guided direct Ganglia neurolysis and block. Am J Gastroenterol 2008;103:98–103. Available at: https://pubmed.ncbi.nlm.nih.gov/17970834/. [Accessed 27 December 2023].

43. Levy MJ, Gleeson FC, Topazian MD, et al. Combined Celiac Ganglia and Plexus Neurolysis Shortens Survival, Without Benefit, vs Plexus Neurolysis Alone. Clin Gastroenterol Hepatol 2019;17:728–38.e9. Available at: https://pubmed.ncbi.nlm.nih.gov/30217513/. [Accessed 27 December 2023].

44. Kaufman M, Singh G, Das S, et al. Efficacy of endoscopic ultrasound-guided celiac plexus block and celiac plexus neurolysis for managing abdominal pain associated with chronic pancreatitis and pancreatic cancer. J Clin Gastroenterol 2010;44:127–34. Available at: https://pubmed.ncbi.nlm.nih.gov/19826273/. [Accessed 27 December 2023].

45. Sey M, Schmaltz L, Al-Haddad M, et al. Effectiveness and safety of serial endoscopic ultrasound-guided celiac plexus block for chronic pancreatitis. Endosc Int Open 2015;3:E56–9. Available at: https://pubmed.ncbi.nlm.nih.gov/26134773/. [Accessed 27 December 2023].

46. Gress F, Schmitt C, Sherman S, et al. Endoscopic ultrasound-guided celiac plexus block for managing abdominal pain associated with chronic pancreatitis: a prospective single center experience. Am J Gastroenterol 2001;96:409–16. Available at: https://pubmed.ncbi.nlm.nih.gov/11232683/. [Accessed 27 December 2023].

47. Gress F, Schmitt C, Sherman S, et al. A Prospective Randomized Comparison of Endoscopic Ultrasound- and Computed Tomography-Guided Celiac Plexus Block for Managing Chronic Pancreatitis Pain. Am J Gastroenterol 1999;94:900–5.

48. Puli SR, Reddy JBK, Bechtold ML, et al. EUS-guided celiac plexus neurolysis for pain due to chronic pancreatitis or pancreatic cancer pain: a meta-analysis and systematic review. Dig Dis Sci 2009;54:2330–7. Available at: https://pubmed.ncbi.nlm.nih.gov/19137428/. [Accessed 27 December 2023].

49. Stevens T, Costanzo A, Lopez R, et al. Adding triamcinolone to endoscopic ultrasound-guided celiac plexus blockade does not reduce pain in patients with chronic pancreatitis. Clin Gastroenterol Hepatol 2012;10. Available at: https://pubmed.ncbi.nlm.nih.gov/21946121/. [Accessed 27 December 2023].

50. Michaels AJ, Draganov PV. Endoscopic ultrasonography guided celiac plexus neurolysis and celiac plexus block in the management of pain due to pancreatic cancer and chronic pancreatitis. World J Gastroenterol 2007;13:3575–80. Available at: https://pubmed.ncbi.nlm.nih.gov/17659707/. [Accessed 27 December 2023].

51. Lillemoe KD, Cameron JL, Kaufman HS, et al. Chemical splanchnicectomy in patients with unresectable pancreatic cancer. A prospective randomized trial. Ann Surg 1993;217:447–57. Available at: https://pubmed.ncbi.nlm.nih.gov/7683868/. [Accessed 27 December 2023].

52. Muscatiello N, Panella C, Pietrini L, et al. Complication of endoscopic ultrasound-guided celiac plexus neurolysis. Endoscopy 2006;38:858. Available at: https://pubmed.ncbi.nlm.nih.gov/17001583/. [Accessed 27 December 2023].

53. HM A, SE F, HF H, et al. End-organ ischemia as an unforeseen complication of endoscopic-ultrasound-guided celiac plexus neurolysis. Endoscopy 2009;

41(Suppl 2):E218–9. Available at: https://pubmed.ncbi.nlm.nih.gov/19757362/. [Accessed 27 December 2023].

54. Jang HY, Cha SW, Lee BH, et al. Hepatic and splenic infarction and bowel ischemia following endoscopic ultrasound-guided celiac plexus neurolysis. Clin Endosc 2013;46:306–9. Available at: https://pubmed.ncbi.nlm.nih.gov/23767046/. [Accessed 27 December 2023].

55. Petersen EW, Pohler KR, Burnett CJ, et al. Pulmonary embolism: a rare complication of neurolytic alcohol celiac plexus block. Pain Physician 2017;20:E751–3. Available at: https://europepmc.org/article/MED/28727720. [Accessed 27 December 2023].

56. Shimizu K, Ito T, Irisawa A, et al. Evidence-based clinical practice guidelines for chronic pancreatitis 2021. J Gastroenterol 2022;57:709–24. Available at: https://pubmed.ncbi.nlm.nih.gov/35994093/. [Accessed 27 December 2023].

57. Singh VK, Yadav D, Garg PK. Diagnosis and Management of Chronic Pancreatitis: A Review. JAMA 2019;322:2422–34. Available at: https://pubmed.ncbi.nlm.nih.gov/31860051/. [Accessed 27 December 2023].

Endoscopic Retrograde Cholangiopancreatography for Management of Chronic Pancreatitis

Aliana Bofill-Garcia, MD*, Camille Lupianez-Merly, MD

KEYWORDS

- Chronic pancreatitis • Endoscopic retrograde cholangiopancreatography
- Pancreatic stones • Pancreatic strictures • Pancreatoscopy-guided lithotripsy
- Extracorporeal shock wave lithotripsy

KEY POINTS

- Endoscopic therapy is the first-line therapeutic approach to pancreatic drainage in chronic pancreatitis (CP) for long-term management of pain.
- Endoscopic retrograde cholangiopancreatography (ERCP) and extracorporeal shock wave lithotripsy (ESWL) are the mainstay therapeutic modalities to manage symptomatic pancreatic duct stones in CP.
- Endoscopic treatment of pancreatic strictures by insertion of pancreatic stents aims to alleviate pain by decompression and remodeling of the stricture.

 Video content accompanies this article at http://www.giendo.theclinics.com.

INTRODUCTION

Chronic pancreatitis (CP) is a persistent pathologic fibroinflammatory syndrome of the pancreas leading to irreversible parenchymal injury and destruction of the functional pancreatic tissue, resulting in permanent loss of function. The most common etiology is alcohol, followed by smoking, and other less common including autoimmune disease, genetic disorders, recurrent acute pancreatitis, obstructive causes, or idiopathic.[1] CP is a debilitating condition with a global incidence of 1.6 to 23 per 100.000 people.[2] The dominant symptom is abdominal pain, with other symptoms such as

Department of Gastroenterology and Hepatology, Mayo Clinic Rochester, 200 First Street Southwest, Rochester, MN 55905, USA
* Corresponding author. Department of Gastroenterology and Hepatology, Mayo Clinic Rochester, Joseph 6-201, 200 First Street Southwest, Rochester, MN 55905.
E-mail address: bofill-garcia.aliana@mayo.edu

Gastrointest Endoscopy Clin N Am 34 (2024) 449–473
https://doi.org/10.1016/j.giec.2024.02.004
1052-5157/24/© 2024 Elsevier Inc. All rights reserved.

exocrine pancreatic insufficiency and endocrine dysfunction developing at variable rates.

The pathophysiology of pain in CP is multifactorial making management often challenging. One of the earliest proposed mechanisms for the development of pain is increased main pancreatic duct (MPD) pressure caused by ductal hypertension, which is suggested to be triggered by increased ductal stretch and parenchymal ischemia secondary to obstruction from stones or stricture. In these cases, decompressing therapies can be attempted to relieve the pain. Additionally, it has been suggested that pain can arise from chronic inflammation and central sensitization by neuropathic changes including structural changes to the intrapancreatic nerves and functional changes in both pancreatic nociceptive neurons and spinal and central neurons.[3,4] Due to its neuropathic involvement, as well as increase narcotic dependence among CP patients, pain may persist or relapse despite endoscopic interventions and MPD decompression.

Abdominal pain is often associated with a lower quality of life (QoL), higher rates of disability, and increased burden to the hospital system and healthcare costs, therefore it is the target for therapy. For decades, management was primarily surgical, however with recent technological advancements and more available endoscopic tools, the management has rapidly evolved to a less invasive approach. This article will focus on standard endoscopic retrograde cholangiopancreatography (ERCP) decompressive techniques for the management of CP complications.

APPROACH TO MANAGEMENT

To determine the best approach to pain management in CP, patients should be evaluated by an interdisciplinary team early in the course of the disease. A pre-interventional evaluation including cross-sectional imaging to tailor the best treatment strategy for the individual patient is crucial. The first step suggested to relieve pain includes lifestyle modifications and pharmacotherapy. Interventional therapy is recommended for patients with refractory pain and characteristics mentioned later in this article. Early studies have suggested that complete resolution of pain was more likely to be achieved from surgery than from endoscopic therapy.[5,6] The ESCAPE trial was a randomized controlled trial (RCT) that compared early surgery versus endoscopy-first approach and replicated these findings.[7] Although these studies have their limitations including the subjectivity of the pain score and no sham-control, data favor that surgical intervention at an earlier stage may help alleviate disease progression, leading to improved pain management, and the preservation of pancreatic function.[7]

A systematic review and meta-analysis concluded that surgical intervention provided long-term pain relief without significant difference in short-term relief when compared to endoscopy. Adverse events (AEs) and length of hospital stay were similar between groups.[8] Although data suggest that surgical interventions are superior to endoscopy for long term management of pain, endoscopic advancements have led societies to favor ERCP and/or extracorporeal shock wave lithotripsy (ESWL) as first-line approach to pancreatic drainage in view of its minimal invasiveness and low AE rate (**Table 1**).[9–12] Surgery should be reserved if endoscopic approaches have been exhausted or unsuccessful. Characteristics suggestive of long-term clinical success with ERCP and/or ESWL include absence of a pancreatic duct (PD) stricture, short disease duration, improved pain (with decreased narcotic use), smoking and alcohol cessation, pancreatic head stones, lack of PD divisum, if stenting was required, and steatorrhea.[10] In addition, patients with inflammatory

Table 1
Society guidelines on endoscopic management of painful uncomplicated chronic pancreatitis with obstructed main pancreatic duct

Society	Endoscopic Management to Relief Pain in Chronic Pancreatitis	Endoscopic Management of Pancreatic Stones	Endoscopic Management of Pancreatic Strictures
ESGE	1st line: ET and/or ESWL with evaluation of clinical response at 6–8 w; if unsatisfactory, discuss in a multidisciplinary team + consider surgery	1st line: ESWL for radiopaque >5 mm head/body stones and ERCP for small <5 mm or radiolucent stones. ERCP following ESWL if no spontaneous clearance of stone fragments. POP-directed lithotripsy when ESWL is not available or for refractory stones after ESWL.	1st line: single 10 Fr PS for 1 uninterrupted year if symptoms improve after initial successful drainage. Stent should be exchanged based on symptoms or signs of stent dysfunction in follow-up imaging every 6 m. Refractory stricture: Multidisciplinary discussion to consider multiple PS. FCSEMSs needs further evaluation due to potential complications.
ASGE	1st line: ET in centers with this expertise, reserving surgery for cases of failure and/or recurrent symptoms.	ESWL + ERCP for symptomatic pancreatolithiasis refractory to standard ERCP techniques.	1st line: ERCP + dilation and/or PS placement after multidisciplinary article considering ET as the preferred initial therapy
ICGCP	Endoscopic or surgical treatment should be offered to patients with CP with persistent severe pain. Intervention is not recommended in asymptomatic patients to improve pancreatic exocrine and/or endocrine function or prevent cancer.	1st line: ESWL for MPD stones who do not get adequate pain relief with conservative management although a stent placement may be done first to relieve pain. ERCP for small stones or stone fragments after ESWL.	1st line: Straight PS across the stricture depending on the caliber of the stricture. Exchange or remove every 2–3 m. Multiple PS vs FCSEMS may be considered for refractory strictures. Surgical intervention for failed endoscopic procedures.
AGA	Surgical intervention > ET for long- term painful obstructive CP. For suboptimal surgical candidates or less invasive approach, ET is a reasonable alternative.	RCP with conventional stone extraction maneuvers for ≤5 mm MPD stones. For larger stones, ESWL and/or pancreatoscopy with intraductal lithotripsy may be required.	Prolonged stent therapy (6–12 m) for symptoms and remodeling MPD strictures. Preferred approach: place and sequentially add MSP in parallel (upsizing). Emerging evidence suggests that FCSEMS may have a role for this indication but additional research is necessary.

(continued on next page)

Table 1
(continued)

Society	Endoscopic Management to Relief Pain in Chronic Pancreatitis	Endoscopic Management of Pancreatic Stones	Endoscopic Management of Pancreatic Strictures
ACG	Surgery > ET in obstructive CP for the long-term relief of pain if first-line endoscopic approaches to pancreatic drainage have been exhausted or unsuccessful.		Sequentially adding MPS in parallel (upsizing) for 6–12 m for symptom treatment and remodeling of the stricture. FCSEMS may have a role for this indication, but additional research is needed.

Abbreviations: ACG, American College of Gastroenterology; AGA, American Gastroenterological Association; ASGE, American Society for Gastrointestinal Endoscopy; CP, chronic pancreatitis; ERCP, endoscopic retrograde cholangiopancreatography; ESGE, European Society of Gastrointestinal Endoscopy; ESWL, extracorporeal shock wave lithotripsy; ET, endoscopic therapy; FCSEMS, fully-covered self-expanding metal stent; ICGP, International Consensus Guidelines on Chronic Pancreatitis; MPD, main pancreatic duct; MPS, multiple plastic stents; PD, pancreatic duct; POP, per oral pancreatoscopy-directed lithotripsy; PS, plastic stent; SEMS, self-expanding metal stents.

masses might be difficult to treat endoscopically.[13] Favorable prognostic factors include complete stone clearance and remodeling of the stricture after stenting.[10]

Pain Characteristics that Require Intervention

- Pain related to large PD disease
- Persistent and continuous pain with or without exacerbations
- Refractory pain to medical treatment
- Pain lasting more than 3 months

ENDOSCOPIC RETROGRADE CHOLANGIOPANCREATOGRAPHY FOR PANCREATIC STONES

Intraductal stones account for 50% of the cases of CP with PD obstruction, 18% by stones alone and 32% by a combination of stones and stricture, with an increase in prevalence over time after disease onset.[14,15] In a multicenter survey of 879 patients with either newly diagnosed or long-standing CP, stones were more frequent in men, heavy drinkers, and heavy smokers.[16] These seem to arise as evenly calcified stones or as radiolucent protein plugs that may or may not become calcified during progression of the disease.[17] The vast majority are calcified and radiopaque, solitary, located in the pancreatic head, with a mean size of 10 mm, and in 50% of the cases are associated with an MPD stricture.[10] Those seen in the nonalcoholic and idiopathic type of CP are usually larger and denser than those seen in the alcohol related type, which are typically small, irregular, and with hazy margins.[18]

Over the course of the last several decades, endoscopic techniques have been the mainstay therapeutic modality to manage symptomatic pancreatic stones (PS) by lowering the intraductal pressure and restoring drainage of the MPD. An increase in ductal pressure that causes pain indicates a dilation of the MPD of greater than 5 mm in diameter.[2] In these selected patients, with marked ductal changes, endoscopic therapy with PD clearance, either with or without ESWL, dilation, and stenting are approaches for PD decompression. This is justified by the belief that endoscopic drainage causes an increase in pancreatic juice flow resulting in a decrease in ductal pressure with relief of pain as a result. However, not all stones can be managed similarly for which selection of the ideal candidate is important to achieve successful treatment and prevention of AEs. In addition, these techniques can be challenging due to underlying MPD strictures and the difference between the size of the stone and the downstream PD.

The success of ERCP-guided treatment is largely influenced by the type, size, number, and location of the stone. In addition, the operator's skill set and the availability of equipment also plays an important role for successful stone clearance. Conventional ERCP with standard techniques including pancreatic sphincterotomy and balloon sphincteroplasty followed by balloon or basket extraction is often reserved for smaller (<5 mm) and radiolucent stones.[10,19] Additionally, patients with less than 3 stones in the head or body with a dilated MPD of greater than 5 mm are better candidates for standard ERCP.[2]

ENDOSCOPIC RETROGRADE CHOLANGIOPANCREATOGRAPHY TECHNIQUE FOR STONE EXTRACTION

Before attempting stone extraction, a pancreatic sphincterotomy is first performed using a sphincterotome over a guidewire. This can be performed at the minor papilla if evidence of pancreas divisum. Subsequently, balloon sphincteroplasty up to 4 to 6 mm can be performed in case of a stricture in the pancreatic head.[2,20,21] After achieving adequate PD access, baskets/balloons can be used to extract the stones. One of the most common AEs is a trapped or broken basket during stone extraction[22],for which balloon has shown to be safer, as they can be detached if trapped.[23] Nonetheless, often these stones sharp edges puncture and destroy both dilation and extraction balloons easily. Other factors associated with failed stone clearance include size greater than 10 mm, diffuse location, underlying downstream stricture, and stone impaction.[24,25]

Larger stones (>5 mm) are often more challenging to extract by standard ERCP only, and in 70% to 90% of the cases additional treatment methods for stone fragmentation is required to facilitate extraction.[19] The reported success rate with the use of Dormia basket is only 9%.[26] Mechanical lithotripsy is often not effective because of the hardness of the stones and also by the challenge of manipulating the larger basket in a tortuous and thin caliber MPD along with impaction of the stone. Due to the higher risk of failure and AEs related to fracture of basket wires and duct injury, it is used less frequently than biliary stone lithotripsy.[22] Lithotripsy is often utilized for fragmentation and options include mechanical lithotripsy, ESWL, and intraductal therapy with pancreatoscopy.

EXTRACORPORAL SHOCK WAVE LITHOTRIPSY FOR PANCREATIC STONES

As an alternative to conventional endoscopy, stone fragmentation with ESWL was introduced. It can be performed with or without subsequent ERCP to clear stone fragments from the PD. ESWL is based on the principle of shock wave energy, initially introduced in the early 1980s for the treatment of urinary stones and a few years later expanded to biliary/pancreatic stones (PS).[27,28] Over the years, studies have supported the use of ESWL and it is currently the cornerstone treatment modality for patients with painful uncomplicated CP and large stones that are not amenable to extraction by standard ERCP.[10,12]

The goal of ESWL is to achieve stone fragmentation to lesser than 3 mm in size or demonstrate a decrease in density of the stone mass.[29] Small fragments can either pass off spontaneously or are extracted with subsequent ERCP. Criteria for technical success of MPD clearance following ESWL are classified as complete (clearance of > 90% of stone volume), partial (clearance 50%–90%), and unsuccessful (<50%). Clinical success is usually based on pain relief, decreased use of pain medication, decreased need for hospitalization, and improvement in QoL. ESWL has been associated with a highly effective stone fragmentation rate with complete clearance rates reported between 70% and 90%[30] and with decreased number of ERCPs required to complete treatment.[30,31]

The first case series of ESWL alone, reported in 1996 from Japan, showed pain relief in 79% of the patients at 3.5 years follow-up.[32] A large prospective single-center series (N = 1006) evaluated ESWL for large PSs not amenable to extraction with ERCP. The stones were fragmented to lesser than 3 mm size and then cleared by endotherapy within 24 to 48 hours with stenting when indicated. The authors observed that 90% of patients needed lesser than 3 sessions of ESWL and at 6 months, 84% had significant pain relief with a decrease in analgesic use.[33] The same group later published one of the largest ESWL studies, which included the 1006 cases reported previously, showing complete stone clearance rate of 72.6% with most of the patients requiring 3 sessions of ESWL and only 4% requiring 5 to 8 sessions to achieve stone clerance.[34] In a more recent meta-analysis of 3868 patients, complete stone fragmentation and ductal clearance was achieved in 86.3% and 69.8% respectively, resulting in absence of pain in over 50%.[35] In studies evaluating relapse, most patients with complete stone clearance who remained pain-free at a 2-year follow-up rarely experienced pain relapse thereafter.[35]

A long-term study of patients with CP undergoing ESWL followed by ERCP demonstrated that after 14 years of follow-up 66% of patients had long-term clinical benefits with decrease in hospitalization rate and delayed impairment in exocrine pancreatic function.[36] Furthermore, this study highlighted the importance of environmental factors such as smoking cessation for achieving superior clinical outcomes. Similar long-term benefits were noted in patients undergoing ESWL combined with ERCP with 60% of patients having absence of abdominal pain more than 60 months after undergoing treatment.[37] Interestingly, most of the patients in this study were young (<40 years old) for which the authors concluded that early intervention, especially in young patients, may alter the course of the disease and possibly prevent the need of surgery in the future.

EXTRACORPORAL SHOCK WAVE LITHOTRIPSY WITH OR WITHOUT ENDOSCOPIC RETROGRADE CHOLANGIOPANCREATOGRAPHY

The use of ERCP following successful and complete fragmentation of stones by ESWL versus ESWL as standalone therapy has been a topic of debate. Studies have shown that if ESWL is performed adequately, the fragments may spontaneously clear obviating the need for ERCP.[32,38] Vaysee and colleagues demonstrated that ERCP did not provide additional benefit compared to ESWL alone.[39] An RCT comparing ESWL alone versus ESWL followed by ERCP demonstrated equal efficacy between the 2 arms, but the cost of the procedure was 3 times higher in patients who underwent both the procedures.[40] The authors concluded that ESWL is safe, but the addition of ERCP added to the cost without improving the outcome of pain control. However, other studies have reported that ESWL alone is not cost effective due to the need for multiple sessions (>10) to ensure adequate fragmentation and spontaneous clearance with an increased risk of impacted stone fragments at risk for pancreatitis.[41,42] In clinical practice, ERCP is routinely performed after ESWL as complete stone clearance is associated with improved abdominal pain. Both the European Society for Gynocological Endoscopy and International consensus guidelines recommend that patients with MPD head/body stones greater than 5 mm should undergo ESWL, followed by ERCP for duct clearance, if there has not been spontaneous clearance after adequate fragmentation.[10,11]

TIMING OF EXTRACORPORAL SHOCK WAVE LITHOTRIPSY WITH ENDOSCOPIC RETROGRADE CHOLANGIOPANCREATOGRAPHY

The optimal timing of ESWL in relation to ERCP is not clearly defined and most institutions that offer ESWL have implemented their own protocols. It has been argued that delaying ERCP after ESWL helps reduce papillary and tissue edema and improves the success of stone clearance.[43] Theoretically, edema around the papilla after ESWL can potentially affect PD cannulation and immediate ERCP after ESWL may cause a "double attack on the pancreas", increasing post-ERCP pancreatitis.[44] Nonetheless, same-day sessions may include faster clearance and relief of abdominal pain, decrease appointments, and travel burden with potential cost savings.[41]

In a small retrospective series, 30 patients were divided between early-ERCP (up to 2 days after ESWL) and delayed-ERCP (>2 days after ESWL) and found that 82% in the delayed group achieved stone clearance compared to 16% in the early group. The authors concluded that timing had a significant impact on the ability to clear the MPD and recommended delaying ERCP to allow tissue recovery.[43] However, this study only included patients who had initially undergone unsuccessful ERCP and required subsequent ESWL. Contradictory results were observed in a retrospective analysis that divided patients in 3 different groups according to the interval time between ESWL and ERCP: lesser than 12 hours, 12 hours to 36 hours, and greater than 36 hours.[44] The authors found that cannulation and stone clearance rates were similarly successful in patients with a history of ERCP, regardless of the timing. However, in those with a native papilla, delaying ERCP improved outcomes, as ESWL can increase the risk of AEs due to difficult cannulation.[44] On the contrary, a recent retrospective study found that delaying ERCP to allow peripancreatic tissue recovery does not affect outcomes and same-day ERCP after ESWL is safe and effective even in those with prior pancreatic sphincterotomy.[41] At the moment, there are no guidelines addressing this issue for which timing is usually left at the discretion of the institution.

SUCCESS, ADVERSE EVENTS, SAFETY, AND LIMITATIONS

Some factors associated with successful endoscopic clearance of stone fragments after ESWL include solitary stones, location at the pancreatic head, density of lesser than 820.5 Hounsfield units on CT scan, secretin injection during the procedure and pre-ESWL pancreatic stent placement.[42,45–49] Other predictive factors include absence of MPD stricture, short disease duration, non-severe pain, and less frequent pancreatitis attacks.[10] These factors may explain the different results between the studies.

ESWL is considered a safe procedure with an overall low AEs rate of 6% to 10% with mild pancreatitis the most common reported.[50,51] Pancreatitis has been reported in up to 4% but it is unclear if it is attributable to the same-day ERCP session[19,34,35] with similar incidence when compared with ESWL plus ERCP versus ERCP alone.[29] Other common AEs include pain and ecchymosis at the site of shockwave, abdominal pain, and fever.[50] Perineal hematoma, biliary obstruction, splenic rupture, bowel perforation, and liver trauma have been rarely reported.[19] Contraindications include non-correctable coagulation disorders, pregnancy, and presence of bone, calcified vessels, or lung tissue in the shockwave path.

Although ESWL is considered standard of care and first-line therapy for large stones, it has some limitations. Failure of stone fragmentation has been reported in approximately 10% of patients with a recurrence of 23% on long-term follow-up.[19,34] Extracorporeal shock wave lithotripsyby itself cannot address concurrent dominant PD strictures, thus additional endoscopic procedures are needed in this setting. In addition, fluoroscopy can detect only radiopaque stones. For radiolucent stones, an intraductal stent prior to ESWL may be placed to target the stones. Other disadvantages include cost, lack of reimbursement, variable efficacy depending on the experience of the operator (most services are provided by urologists), and limited availability in the United States (U.S), impacting generalizability of this approach. Extracorporeal shock wave lithotripsyshould be avoided in patients with extensive calculi involving multiple PD areas, presence of moderate/severe ascites, and suspected pancreatic head mass.[29] Stones in the tail of the pancreas are usually avoided due to risk of splenic rupture.[52]

PER-ORAL PANCREATOSCOPY

Per-oral pancreatoscopy (POP) with intraductal lithotripsy has emerged in recent years as a safe therapeutic alternative for the endoscopic management of PSs. POP has been available since the 1990s, but never gained widespread acceptance due to the technical difficulties, the requirement for 2 operators, and poor imaging quality.[50] With the introduction of the single operator cholangiopancreatoscopy system (SOCP) (SpyGlass DVS; Boston Scientific) in 2007, some of these problems were elucidated but still was underutilized due to suboptimal fiber optic imaging.[53] Later, in 2015, this system was upgraded to a digital version (SpyGlass DS; Boston Scientific) with a 60% wider field of vision, a larger working channel (13 mm), specialized irrigation channel, and improved image quality. Pancreatoscopy-guided lithotripsy (PGL) has been suggested as an alternative to ESWL for PD stones that are refractory to conventional ERCP and/or when ESWL is not available.

PER-ORAL PANCREATOSCOPY-GUIDED FRAGMENTATION SYSTEMS

Pancreatoscopy-guided lithotripsy uses 2 different intraductal fragmentation techniques, electrohydraulic lithotripsy (EHL) and laser lithotripsy (LL), both with different mechanisms of action. EHL consists of a charge generator and a bipolar probe that produces a spark at its tip in an aqueous solution. The sparks produce vapor plasma and subsequently an oscillating cavitating bubble, generating high-amplitude hydraulic pressure waves, which are absorbed by the stones resulting in their fragmentation. In LL, laser light of a specific wavelength is concentrated on the stone's surface to produce wave-mediated fragmentation. The neodymium: yttrium-aluminum-garnet (Nd: YAG) laser breaks stones through the initial formation of plasma on the stone surface which subsequently absorbs the infrared light energy powerfully and generates a strong shockwave. The holmium: YAG laser lithotripsy occurs primarily by a photothermal mechanism where energy is directly transmitted from the laser to the stone.[54] In both mechanisms, the probe needs to be directed at the stone at a distance of greater than or equal to 5 mm without making contact. If the probe is not deployed near the stone and away from the duct wall, the shock waves may induce damage or even perforation to the wall.[55]

PER-ORAL PANCREATOSCOPY-GUIDED LITHOTRIPSY TECHNIQUE

The pancreatoscope has a small diameter (3.3 mm/10 Fr) and can be introduced through the working channel of a duodenoscope. It has its own working channel, through which accessories (minimum diameter 1.2 mm/3.2 Fr) can be introduced. When performing PGL, a pancreatic sphincterotomy and/or a sphincteroplasty of 4 mm are necessary to enter the MPD.[2] Once deep wire access is obtained, the pancreatoscope can be advanced to the stone, the guidewire removed, and lithotripsy is performed under direct vision. Stone fragments can be then removed with standard ERCP techniques including balloon sweep and basket retrieval. If a stricture is encountered downstream to the stone, a step-up-dilation up to 10 Fr should be performed prior to attempting POP.[2] It has been suggested that after PGL, a PS (9–10 Fr) should be placed if there is an underlying stricture.[56] Saline irrigation should be reduced to a necessary minimum and the patient should receive nonsteroidal anti-inflammatory suppositories and intravenous hydration as high pressure in the MPD can increase the risk of post-ERCP pancreatitis (PEP).[56] In addition, prophylactic antibiotic use is recommended in all cases due to risk of systemic bacterial translocation during saline irrigation.[55] Video 1 shows a case of effective PD stone fragmentation with EHL.

PER-ORAL PANCREATOSCOPY-GUIDED LITHOTRIPSY OUTCOMES

In recent years, several retrospective studies have demonstrated a stone clearance rate ranging from 43% to 100% with recent larger studies showing rates between 80% and 90%.[50,51,57–60] This variability can be explained by the retrospective designs of the studies, small sample sizes, short follow-up, and varied patient selection and treatment protocols. In a retrospective review, patients who underwent ERCP with POP had higher technical success than those with ERCP alone (n = 129, 98.9% vs 87.6%, P < .001), but required more ERCPs (3.1 vs 1.9). ERCP with POP was associated with larger stone size (8.9 vs 6.1 mm, P = .001), more stones per case, and more impacted stones.[61]

In a meta-analysis that included 16 studies, the overall technical and clinical success rates were 76% and 77% respectively. Factors influencing lower technical success included multiple or impacted stones, size greater than 17 mm, strictures, difficulty in cannulating the PD due to angulation, poor visibility, and equipment failure.[62] On direct comparative analysis, LL had higher overall rates of technical and clinical success with comparable AE rates and less procedure time.[62] The advantage theoretically was explained by the ability of LL to fragment denser stones. The presence of 3 or more stones has been reported as a significant independent risk for failure of PGL.[50] Contrary, increased stone burden has led to higher technical success rates as these patients had higher probabilities of having smaller stones which are easier to clear compared to larger stones.[61]

Conversely, a meta-analysis evaluating POP with either LL or EHL for the treatment of difficult PD stones defined as failure of conventional ERCP, showed high technical success rates (91%) but no significant difference between EHL and LL.[63] Currently, there is no comparative study evaluating which of these 2 techniques is more effective in pancreatic stone fragmentation. In most of the studies, POP was performed after unsuccessful stone fragmentation with standard ERCP and in some ESWL, highlighting POP as an alternative option when first-line therapies fail.[62,63] However, can this be a promising first-line treatment for CP patients with obstructive stones? In a prospective, single-center study evaluating the efficacy and safety of EHL as a first-line treatment for stones in the head/neck of the pancreas, authors reported a technical success rate of 70.6%, which was mainly limited by the inability to achieve deep cannulation of the PD. When POP was successful, the success rate increased to 92.3% with complete stone removal in 80% of the patients with a median of 2 ERCP and 1 EHL procedure. Clinical success was achieved in 72% of the patients, with greater than 50% pain score and opioid use reduction over a 6-month follow-up period.[64] However, there was a trend towards higher pain scores and more opiate use at 6 months, suggesting that its benefit may not be long-lasting. A recent prospective multicenter trial also demonstrated high technical success rates (92%) with persistent stone clearance and pain-relief (82%) at 6 month follow-up.[56] However, this data must be carefully interpreted and might not represent both lithotripsy techniques, as only 1 patient underwent LL while the rest underwent EHL. A retrospective 4 center study evaluated LL for PD stones in 28 patients who underwent 1 to 4 POP-LL sessions. Prior history of ESWL or EHL not excluded. The authors demonstrated a total stone clearance of 79% and a clinical success rate of 89% at a median of 13 months with improvement in pain, decreased narcotic use, or reduced hospitalizations. It was concluded that LL could complete stone clearance but at least 1 subsequent PGL or ERCP is needed for additional stone extraction and/or stricture therapy.[57] More prospective studies are needed to assess direct comparison and cost-effective analysis when POP is undertaken.

PER-ORAL PANCREATOSCOPY-GUIDED LITHOTRIPSY ADVANTAGES, ADVERSE EVENTS

Although studies are still sparse, one of the advantages of PGL is direct stone visualization, facilitating precise fragmentation, and confirming clearance of the PD. In addition, concomitant strictures can be assessed and combined with other interventions including stricture dilation, and/or stenting in a single session. Although direct visualization can reduce duct injury, it is important to avoid long periods of PD exposure to high energy levels in a single session, given the risk of thermal injury to the duct wall. Some of the limitations include significant costs, the need for device expertise to achieve cannulation, as well as the need for longer procedure durations, and moderate success rates when compared to conventional strategies.[63] Additionally, the success of a pancreatoscopy will largely depend by the MPD anatomy, strictures, or obstructing stones. For cephalic stones, PGL could be challenging due to device instability and/or difficulty visualization. Compared to standard ERCP or ESWL, PGL is more technically challenging as it is often difficult to advance the pancreatoscope catheter even in a normal caliber PD with some authors suggesting that an MPD diameter of 4 to 5 mm is necessary to allow passage.[55] Compared to EHL, LL is more expensive, needs special precautions, and the equipment is less compact.[62] The overall AE rates after PGL have been reported at 10% to 12%[10,60] and mostly consisted of mild pancreatitis; similar findings when compared to ESWL.

Although PGL appears to be effective, its precise role in the treatment of difficult stones remains unclear. Upcoming devices suitable for the single-operator cholangiopancreatoscopy could open new additional option for therapeutic procedures. Currently there are no standardized protocols or treatment strategies, thus more studies are needed to validate its role in the therapeutic algorithm of CP. However, according to available studies and societies recommendations, PD stones in CP can be managed as suggested in the algorithm illustrated in **Fig. 1**.

MAIN PANCREATIC DUCT STRICTURES

Benign strictures of the MPD occur in CP because of inflammation and/or fibrosis. They can present as single or multiple and classified as dominant, or nondominant.

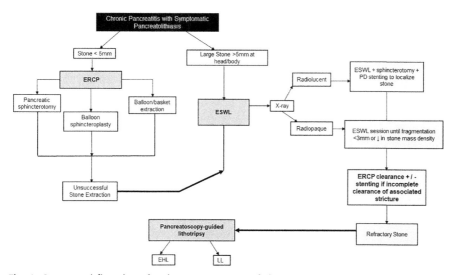

Fig. 1. Suggested flowchart for the management of chronic pancreatitis with symptomatic pancreatolithiasis. EHL, electrohydraulic lithotripsy; ERCP, endoscopic retrograde cholangiopancreatography; ESWL, extracorporeal shock wave lithotripsy; LL, laser lithotripsy; PD pancreatic duct.

Dominant strictures are associated with upstream MPD dilation and often lead to pain and superimposed acute on CP. Endoscopic treatment of PD strictures by insertion of pancreatic stents aims to alleviate pain by decompression and steadily stricture dilation to a size that will allow stent removal without recurrence. Long-term clinical success is achieved when the patient remains pain free during the year following stent removal. Technical success has been defined as successful stent insertion across a dominant MPD stricture or the most distal (tail) stricture when multiple strictures are present.[10] Studies have reported a technical success rate of 90% of a first stent insertion.[6,65,66] Nonetheless, these strictures are often tight and difficult to treat for which dilation prior to stenting is recommended, relieving abdominal pain in more than 50% of patients.[65] **Fig. 2** illustrates a case of a severe head/neck PD stricture where dilation was performed prior to stenting.

A greater extent of dilation and stricture remodeling can be achieved by upsizing the caliber of the stent or by sequential placement of multiple side-by-side plastic stents (PS).[67,68] However, this requires multiple interventions, as durable stricture remodeling usually takes up 6 to 12 months of incremental replacement and upsizing of stents. Refractory strictures, defined as symptomatic dominant strictures that persist or relapse after greater than 1 year of single 10 Fr stent insertion,[10] may be treated by multiple side-by-side PS or self-expandable metal stents (SEMS).[69]

For pancreatic stenting to be successful, it is paramount to understand the cause of the stricture, as well as to evaluate the anatomy with dedicated pancreatic imaging. If the etiology of the stricture is not evident, excluding malignancy with cytology brushing should be initially performed.[12] Some of the PD stricture studies discussed later are summarized in **Table 2**.

SINGLE PLASTIC STENTS

Insertion of a single PS has been used as the initial endoscopic therapy for symptomatic MPD stricture caused by CP.[10] Several stenting designs have been proposed, including, straight, curved, wedge or single pigtail but, the presence of side holes to allow drainage of side branches are the distinguishing feature of dedicated pancreatic stents. Their ends also vary with 1 or 2 internal flanges to prevent migration and 2 external flanges or pigtail to prevent inward migration.[70] To improve pancreatic stenting, a nonflanged, multi-fenestrated PS with an ultra-tapered tip (Johlin Wedge Stent; Cook Medical, Winston-Salem, NC) was developed. These are made of a soft polymer blend material that minimizes injury by the tip and can be customized per patient to a

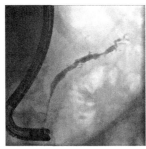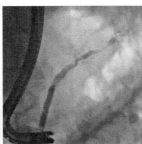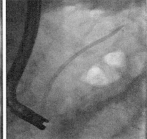

Fig. 2. Pancreatogram with evidence of severe chronic pancreatitis, classified as Cambridge grade 5. Notable stricture in the pancreas head. Ballon dilation to 6 mm of the strictured portion of the MPD followed by the placement of a 10 Fr PS across the stricture. MPD, main pancreatic duct; PS, plastic stent.

Table 2
Key studies comparing the different modalities and types of stents for MPD strictures in CP

Type of Stent	Patient Group	Type of Study	Stent Duration (m)	Key Findings			Complications	Comments	Related Study
				Long-Term Outcomes	Median Follow-up	Pain Relief			
PS vs surgery	Painful CP with MPD strictures predominantly head/body. N = 140 Randomization: 76 underwent surgery 64 treated endoscopically 33/64 stented	Prospective	16 (exchange every 2–4)	Technical success: 62/64 (97%)	5 y	Complete or partial pain relief at 5 follow-up in 65% (of 64 ET patients) ↓ Melzack score	Post-ERCP complications: 5/64 (8%) bleeding: 2 pancreatitis:2 pancreatic abscess: 1 mortality: 0	Pseudo-randomization High bias risk Not an ITT analysis.	Dite et al,[5] 2003
Johlin-JPWS® stent (Cook®)	Painful CP N = 13	Retrospective	4.5 ± 3 (0.5–3.5)	91% clinical success rate at the end of follow-up	11 ± 7 m (1.5–24)	11/13 patients ↓analgesic +/–reduction in the frequency of pain	Uncomplicated acute pancreatitis (10%) No stent migration		Boursier et al,[71] 2008
Single PS temporary pancreatic stenting vs non-stenting	Severe CP with dominant MPD stricture Stenting: N = 20 Non-stenting: N = 22	Prospective, non-randomized	15.2 (exchange every 2–3)	Re-stenting: 2/20 vs 3/22	5.2 y	Pain relapses: Stenting: 3/20 Non-stenting: 11/22	NA		Seza et al,[65] 2011

(continued on next page)

Table 2
(continued)

Type of Stent	Patient Group	Type of Study	Stent Duration (m)	Key Findings				Comments	Related Study
				Long-Term Outcomes	Median Follow-up	Pain Relief	Complications		
MPS after single PS refractory stricture	Severe CP requiring pancreatic stenting N = 19	Prospective	7 (5–11)	84% asymptomatic at 38 m mean follow-up	38 m (17–55)	Symptom-free period: longer after removal of MPS than by single PS	10.5% symptom recurrence	First study to assess the placement of MPS within the PD for CP dominant strictures in the head of the pancreas	Costamagna et al,[68] 2006
Multiple vs SPS	Painful CP and distal MPD obstruction N = 85 Divided in 3 groups: A: exclusively one stent B: 1 or 2 PS C: 2 PS during the stenting period	Observational	A:14.5 (9–27) B:23 (16–33) C: 22.5 (15–31)	Median procedures A: 3 (1–3) B: 4 (3–5) C: 3 (2–3) Clinical success: Group C:50% Group A:88.2% Group B:74.2%	89 m (64–108)	Refractory stricture with MPS: pain recurrence after PS:10 patients (29%)	Stent migration: A: 3 (17%) B:9 (26%) C: 6 (19%) post-ERCP pancreatitis: 2 duodenal perforation: 1	Initial single stenting deployment was associated with a higher rate of clinical success compared to patients with initial placement of 2 stents.	Papalavrentios et al,[101] 2019
MPS after refractory PS	CP and refractory single PS N = 48	Retrospective analysis of a previous prospective study	6.8 (6–18)	83.3% MPD stricture resolution after stent removal 100% refractory strictures re-treated and 37.5% cured	9.5 y (0.3–15.5)	74.4% remained asymptomatic after initial stricture resolution	Pancreatitis recurrence or pancreatitis type pain: 25% Refractory stricture:10.4%		Tringali et al,[67] 2019

Indication	Population	Study design		Outcome	Follow-up	Pain	Complications	Limitations	Reference
FCSEMS (sustained response after removal)	CP strictures refractory to PS N = 6	Prospective	3 (87–100 d)	Recurrent PD stricture in 3/5 patients after 1-and 4-m post removal	4 w after stent removal	>50% pain relapse after stent removal, which later resolved after re-stenting for 3 m	No complications reported	Limitations: Pilot study	Sauer et al,[86] 2008
FCSEMS for refractory PD strictures	Previously drained stents for CP N = 33	Retrospective Multicenter (USA experience case series)	14	Recurrence rate 0% in 8 m	8 m	Using VAS pain score:87.1% significant pain reduction with reduced narcotic use	Cholestasis after stent placement: 6.06% Worsening abdominal pain: 8.2%		Sharaiha et al,[100] 2019
Investigational 4- 6-cm-long soft pancreatic FC-SEMS	CP with PS placement within 90 d of FCSEMS N = 67	Prospective, multicenter	6	Clinical success rate: 6.1%	6 months after FC-SEMS removal	Pain reduction 6 mo after FC-SEMS: 26.1%	Procedure-related SAEs occurred in 31.3% (21/67) Study stent migrations occurred in 47.7% (31/65)	Clinical success rate was lower than the performance goal set for the study (53%)	Sherman et al,[85] 2023
FCSEMS vs PS	CP with persistent MPD strictures after SPS N = 80 FCSEMS N = 26 PS N = 54	Retrospective	FCSEMS: up to 6 m PS- 3–6 m	MPD stricture resolution rate: FC-SEMS: 87% PS: 42%	FCSEMS: 33.7 m PS: 36.2 m	Using VAS pain score: FCSEMS: 76.9 PS: 53.7	Spontaneous stent migration FCSEMS: 26.9% PS: 3.7%	FCSEMS had favorable clinical efficacy (pain relief), but > spontaneous migration 1and de novo strictures	Lee SH, Kim YS et al,[79] 2021

(continued on next page)

Table 2
(continued)

Type of Stent	Patient Group	Type of Study	Stent Duration (m)	Long-Term Outcomes	Median Follow-up	Pain Relief	Complications	Comments	Related Study
					Key Findings				
MPS vs FCSEMS	106 MPS vs 192 FCSEMS patients from 13 studies refractory to single PS	SRMA	Mean range for SEMS: 2–7 for MPS: 6.6–23.7	Weighted pool rates (WPR) for pain recurrence after MPS: 11.8% after SEMS: 14.8%	Mean range between 5.5–34 m between studies	WPR of pain improvement resolution after SEMS: 88% after MPS: 89%	Risk of stent migration was higher with FCSEMS	Meta-analysis for safety and efficacy did not show any advantage of SEMS over MPS in refractory PD strictures Limitations: all studies were observational, increasing risk of bias	Sofi et al,[80] 2021

Abbreviations: CP, chronic pancreatitis; ET, endoscopic therapy; FCSEMS, fully-covered self-expanding metal stent, ITT, intention-to-treat; mo, months; MPD, main pancreatic duct; MPS, multiple plastic stents; PD, pancreatic duct; PS, plastic stent; SAEs, severe adverse events; SEMS, self-expanding metal stents; SRMA, systematic review and meta-analysis.

length of less than or equal to 22 cm. A single-center retrospective study by Boursier and colleagues evaluated this stent and concluded that it is effective for the immediate and medium-term pain relief and may result in less frequent replacements.[71] The deployment of PS is like biliary stents and whether a pancreatic sphincterotomy should be performed has not been addressed but it should be considered when placing larger caliber stents (>8.5 Fr).[10,70]

Current guidelines recommended index placement of a single 10 Fr PS for 1 uninterrupted year.[10,12] In a retrospective study, patients who were treated with lesser than 8.5 Fr stents were more likely to be hospitalized for abdominal pain than those who received 10 Fr stents.[72] Stents can be exchanged until stricture resolution in a regular time interval or an as-needed basis according to clinical manifestations or suggestion of stent malfunction.[10] In clinical practice most centers favor a regular stent exchange after 3 month as previous studies showed less septic complications when compared to "on-demand" stent exchange or longer intervals.[5,65,66,71,73–77] At this time, a new stent should be inserted if the stricture remains significant.

MULTIPLE SIDE-BY-SIDE PLASTIC STENTS

For refractory strictures, placement of multiple plastic stents (MPS) can be considered. This technique can avoid blockage of a side-branches compared to a single large caliber stent. In a study of 19 patients with refractory strictures, a median of 3 PS were placed and removed after 6 to 12 months. During a mean follow-up of 38 months after stent removal, 84% of patients were asymptomatic, and 10.5% had symptomatic recurrences. The authors concluded that this approach allows for shorter resolution time with fewer stent exchanges.[68] More recently, the same group re-evaluated the long-term results in 48 patients with 89.5% achieving stricture resolution after a single session and 77.1% pain relief during a mean follow-up of 9.5 years.[67]

SELF-EXPANDABLE METAL STENTS

The use of fully covered self-expandable metal stent (FCSEMS) of 6mm-10 mm in diameter as a treatment option for refractory PD strictures has been of recent interest. Currently, none are approved by the U.S. Food and Drug Administration for the PD and most of the U.S and Europe studies have typically used off-label biliary FCSEMS. A meta-analysis including 10 studies with 163 patients treated with FCSEMSs showed a stricture resolution rate of 93% with a recurrence rate of 5%.[78] Similarly, a retrospective study of patients with persistent PD strictures after at least 3 months of initial single PS, showed that FCSEMSs had statistically higher stricture resolution rate compared to PS, but with higher AEs such as spontaneous migration and de novo strictures.[79] A recent systematic article and meta-analysis that compared FCSEMSs and MPS found no differences in pain improvement or stricture recurrence, and like prior studies, it showed higher rate of serious AEs with FCSEMSs.[80]

Several studies from Asia have used PD-specific 6-10 mm FCSEMSs that are more flexible with antimigration features.[81–84] In a long-term study using this type of stent, for refractory strictures, 23% patients experienced recurrence during the 11-year follow-up with a median time to recurrence of 2 years.[84] A novel short, saddle-shaped stent (BONASTENT M-intraductal; Standard Sci Tech Inc, Seoul, South Korea) was developed for targeted intraductal placement and easy retrieval by a lasso attached to the duodenal end.[82] In 25 patients treated with this stent, 100% achieved stricture resolution with only 2 patients developing recurrence at a median follow-up of 24 months following stent removal.[82] On the contrary, in a prospective multicenter study of 67 patients treated with a 4-cm to 6-cm-long soft pancreatic FCSEMS, only 26.1% achieved complete or partial pain relief by 6 months after stent removal and almost half of patients experienced stent migration.[85]

Duration of placement and exchange intervals are still unclear. A study by Sauer and colleagues, found that more than 50% of patients had pain relapse after FCSEMS removal, that later resolved after placement of another one for an additional 3 months.[86] Although studies are promising, prospective studies are needed to evaluate optimal patient selection, as well as long-term efficacy and safety, since most studies have used off-label biliary FCSEMS.

ADVERSE EVENTS OF ENDOSCOPIC PANCREATIC STENT THERAPY

The most common AEs associated with PS are pancreatitis and worsening abdominal pain with an average occurrence of 6%-10%, followed by sepsis, cholangitis, and post-sphincterotomy bleeding.[10,70] Severe pancreatitis is rarely documented. Stent migration, stent occlusion, and stent-induced strictures have also been reported. Proximal and distal migration have been reported in 2.7% and 3.6% of patients, respectively.[87] PD stenting can induce duct changes, including de novo strictures reported in up to 27% of patients who underwent stenting prophylactically (though many of these patients had a normal pancreas).[10,88] Higher rates of de novo-strictures have been reported with FCSEMS, likely related to their flared ends inducing ischemic injury from excessive compression of the MPD due to outward radial forces.[10,70,84]

BENIGN BILIARY STRICTURES

Benign biliary strictures (BBS) have been reported in 3%-46% of patients with CP.[89–91] The incidence may be higher as many of the cases remain asymptomatic. CP-related BBSs are often seen late in the course of the disease as progressive, irreversible pancreatic parenchymal fibrosis leads to stricturing of the distal bile duct. A study of 2153 CP patients aimed to develop a prognostic nomogram for BBS in CP patients. They found that some risk factors associated with the development of these strictures included smoking, MPD morphology, male gender, body mass index, and age of onset of CP, with the latter two and type of pain identified as risk factors for symptomatic strictures.[92] BBS can be present with asymptomatic elevation of liver functions test, jaundice, abdominal pain, and cholangitis.

ERCP for bile duct drainage is recommended in patients presenting with jaundice and subclinical cholestasis for greater than 1 month to prevent the development of secondary biliary cirrhosis. However, the data supporting the latter are notably absent. ERCP with stent placement is considered first-line therapy, unless the patient has a pancreatic head mass suspicious for malignancy[89,93] or if there is no resolution after 1 year or 3 sessions of endotherapy.[10] It is important to keep in mind that transient biliary obstruction can occur secondary to acute inflammation in the setting of edema from acute on CP. However, this usually resolves without specific treatment and does not require intervention.[94] Cholangitis is rare but can occur especially if history of previous biliary sphincterotomy and warrants urgent biliary drainage.[89]

Due to the fibrotic nature of BBS-related to CP, MPS are preferred over a single PS as it can provide gradual remodeling of fibrotic tissue.[95] However, if feasible, FCSEMS are recommended over MSP as they provide similar efficacy without the frequent need for stent exchange.[9,96,97] Currently, only 1 stent (WallFlex stent Boston Scientific) is FDA-approved with a 12-month dwell time for treatment of CP-related BBS. In a multicenter RCT, patients treated with FCSEMS for 12 months had similar stricture resolution rates compared with MPS (76% vs 77% respectively) but required significantly less reinterventions over 24 months.[98] A prospective study evaluating the long-term success and safety of FCSEMS showed that nearly 60% of the patients remain asymptomatic and stent free for up to 5 years after 1 FCSEMS was placed for 10 to 12 months. Severe CP and longer stricture length were identified as predictors of treatment failure.[99] From the data available, placement of a single FCSEMS should be considered as the first-line treatment in BBS related to CP.

CLINICS CARE POINTS

- Pain is the main indication for endoscopic therapy in CP, and in case of intraductal stones and/or strictures, endoscopic treatment can help reduce the intraductal pressure by restoring a sufficient drainage of the MPD.
- Standard ERCP with sphincterotomy, downstream stricture dilation, and balloon and/or basket retrieval may remove small stones but up to 50% of stones will be refractory to this approach.
- Extracorporeal shock wave lithotripsy is the standard of care for managing large stones (>5 mm) and those not amenable to extraction by standard techniques.
- Pancreatoscopy-guided lithotripsy using EHL or LL is a useful tool in treating ductal obstruction with a relatively higher success in cases not amenable to ERCP techniques or failure to ESWL but, more data are needed for better definition of indications and role in the current algorithms.
- Pancreatoscopy-guided lithotripsy can also be paired with an additional intervention, such as PD stricture dilatation and/or PD stenting, in a single session.
- For PD strictures, guidelines recommended index placement of a single 10 Fr PS for 1 uninterrupted year.
- For refractory strictures, MPS or FCSEMS have shown similar clinical and technical success rates, but higher risk of stent migration and de novo strictures with FCSEMS.
- ERCP with stenting in distal biliary strictures related to CP is recommended in patients presenting with jaundice and subclinical cholestasis to prevent the development of secondary biliary cirrhosis.

DISCLOSURE

The authors have nothing to disclose.

SUPPLEMENTARY DATA

Supplementary data to this article can be found online at https://doi.org/10.1016/j.giec.2024.02.004.

REFERENCES

1. Cohen SM, Kent TS. Etiology, Diagnosis, and Modern Management of Chronic Pancreatitis: A Systematic Review. JAMA Surg 2023;158(6):652–61.
2. Gerges C, Beyna T, Neuhaus H. Management of Pancreatic Duct Stones: Non-extracorporeal Approach. Gastrointest Endosc Clin N Am 2023;33(4):821–9.
3. Drewes AM, Bouwense SAW, Campbell CM, et al. Guidelines for the understanding and management of pain in chronic pancreatitis. Pancreatology Sep-Oct 2017;17(5):720–31.

4. Pham A, Forsmark C. Chronic pancreatitis: review and update of etiology, risk factors, and management. F1000Res 2018;7. https://doi.org/10.12688/f1000research.12852.1.

5. Díte P, Ruzicka M, Zboril V, et al. A prospective, randomized trial comparing endoscopic and surgical therapy for chronic pancreatitis. Endoscopy 2003; 35(7):553–8.

6. Cahen DL, Gouma DJ, Laramée P, et al. Long-term outcomes of endoscopic vs surgical drainage of the pancreatic duct in patients with chronic pancreatitis. Gastroenterology 2011;141(5):1690–5.

7. Issa Y, Kempeneers MA, Bruno MJ, et al. Effect of Early Surgery vs Endoscopy-First Approach on Pain in Patients With Chronic Pancreatitis: The ESCAPE Randomized Clinical Trial. JAMA 21 2020;323(3):237–47.

8. Mendieta PJO, Sagae VMT, Ribeiro IB, et al. Pain relief in chronic pancreatitis: endoscopic or surgical treatment? a systematic review with meta-analysis. Surg Endosc 2021;35(8):4085–94.

9. Strand DS, Law RJ, Yang D, et al. AGA Clinical Practice Update on the Endoscopic Approach to Recurrent Acute and Chronic Pancreatitis: Expert Review. Gastroenterology 2022;163(4):1107–14.

10. Dumonceau JM, Delhaye M, Tringali A, et al. Endoscopic treatment of chronic pancreatitis: European Society of Gastrointestinal Endoscopy (ESGE) Guideline - Updated August 2018. Endoscopy 2019;51(2):179–93.

11. Kitano M, Gress TM, Garg PK, et al. International consensus guidelines on interventional endoscopy in chronic pancreatitis. Recommendations from the working group for the international consensus guidelines for chronic pancreatitis in collaboration with the International Association of Pancreatology, the American Pancreatic Association, the Japan Pancreas Society, and European Pancreatic Club. Pancreatology 2020;20(6):1045–55.

12. Committee ASoP, Chandrasekhara V, Chathadi KV, et al. The role of endoscopy in benign pancreatic disease. Gastrointest Endosc 2015;82(2):203–14.

13. Beyer G, Habtezion A, Werner J, et al. Chronic pancreatitis. Lancet 2020; 396(10249):499–512.

14. Rösch T, Daniel S, Scholz M, et al. Endoscopic treatment of chronic pancreatitis: a multicenter study of 1000 patients with long-term follow-up. Endoscopy 2002; 34(10):765–71.

15. Dirweesh A, Trikudanathan G, Freeman ML. Endoscopic Management of Complications in Chronic Pancreatitis. Dig Dis Sci 2022;67(5):1624–34.

16. Frulloni L, Gabbrielli A, Pezzilli R, et al. Chronic pancreatitis: report from a multicenter Italian survey (PanCroInfAISP) on 893 patients. Dig Liver Dis 2009;41(4): 311–7.

17. Sarles H, Camarena J, Gomez-Santana C. Radiolucent and calcified pancreatic lithiasis: two different diseases. Role of alcohol and heredity. Scand J Gastroenterol 1992;27(1):71–6.

18. Chari S, Jayanthi V, Mohan V, et al. Radiological appearance of pancreatic calculi in tropical versus alcoholic chronic pancreatitis. J Gastroenterol Hepatol 1992;7(1):42–4.

19. Tandan M, Talukdar R, Reddy DN. Management of Pancreatic Calculi: An Update. Gut Liver 2016;10(6):873–80.

20. Kim YH, Jang SI, Rhee K, et al. Endoscopic treatment of pancreatic calculi. Clin Endosc 2014;47(3):227–35.

21. Gerges C, Albers D, Schmitz L, et al. Correction: Digital single-operator pancreatoscopy for the treatment of symptomatic pancreatic duct stones: a prospective multicenter cohort trial. Endoscopy 2023;55(2):C1.

22. Thomas M, Howell DA, Carr-Locke D, et al. Mechanical lithotripsy of pancreatic and biliary stones: complications and available treatment options collected from expert centers. Am J Gastroenterol 2007;102(9):1896–902.

23. Committee AT, Adler DG, Conway JD, et al. Biliary and pancreatic stone extraction devices. Gastrointest Endosc 2009;70(4):603–9.

24. Sherman S, Lehman GA, Hawes RH, et al. Pancreatic ductal stones: frequency of successful endoscopic removal and improvement in symptoms. Gastrointest Endosc 1991;37(5):511–7.

25. Suzuki Y, Sugiyama M, Inui K, et al. Management for pancreatolithiasis: a Japanese multicenter study. Pancreas 2013;42(4):584–8.

26. Farnbacher MJ, Schoen C, Rabenstein T, et al. Pancreatic duct stones in chronic pancreatitis: criteria for treatment intensity and success. Gastrointest Endosc 2002;56(4):501–6.

27. Chaussy C, Schmiedt E, Jocham D, et al. First clinical experience with extracorporeally induced destruction of kidney stones by shock waves. J Urol 1982; 127(3):417–20.

28. Sauerbruch T, Stern M. Fragmentation of bile duct stones by extracorporeal shock waves. A new approach to biliary calculi after failure of routine endoscopic measures. Gastroenterology 1989;96(1):146–52.

29. Manu T, Partha P, Duvvuru Nageshwar R. Management of Pancreatic Duct Stones: Extracorporeal Approach. Gastrointestinal Endoscopy Clinics of North America 2023;33(4):807–20.

30. Nguyen-Tang T, Dumonceau JM. Endoscopic treatment in chronic pancreatitis, timing, duration and type of intervention. Best Pract Res Clin Gastroenterol 2010;24(3):281–98.

31. Dumonceau JM, Delhaye M, Cremer M. Extracorporeal shock-wave lithotripsy for gallstone ileus. Gastrointest Endosc 1996;44(6):759.

32. Ohara H, Hoshino M, Hayakawa T, et al. Single application extracorporeal shock wave lithotripsy is the first choice for patients with pancreatic duct stones. Am J Gastroenterol 1996;91(7):1388–94.

33. Tandan M, Reddy DN, Santosh D, et al. Extracorporeal shock wave lithotripsy and endotherapy for pancreatic calculi-a large single center experience. Indian J Gastroenterol 2010;29(4):143–8.

34. Manu T D, Rupjyoti T, Talukdar R, et al. ESWL for large pancreatic calculi: Report of over 5000 patients. Pancreatology 2019;19(7):916–21.

35. van Huijgevoort NCM, Veld JV, Fockens P, et al. Success of extracorporeal shock wave lithotripsy and ERCP in symptomatic pancreatic duct stones: a systematic review and meta-analysis. Endosc Int Open 2020/07/21 2020;08(08): E1070–85.

36. Delhaye M, Arvanitakis M, Verset G, et al. Long-term clinical outcome after endoscopic pancreatic ductal drainage for patients with painful chronic pancreatitis. Clin Gastroenterol Hepatol 2004;2(12):1096–106.

37. Tandan M, Nageshwar Reddy D. Endotherapy in chronic pancreatitis. World J Gastroenterol 2013;19(37):6156–64.

38. Inui K, Tazuma S, Yamaguchi T, et al. Treatment of pancreatic stones with extracorporeal shock wave lithotripsy: results of a multicenter survey. Pancreas 2005; 30(1):26–30.

39. Vaysse T, Boytchev I, Antoni G, et al. Efficacy and safety of extracorporeal shock wave lithotripsy for chronic pancreatitis. Scand J Gastroenterol 2016;51(11): 1380–5.
40. Dumonceau JM, Costamagna G, Tringali A, et al. Treatment for painful calcified chronic pancreatitis: extracorporeal shock wave lithotripsy versus endoscopic treatment: a randomised controlled trial. Gut 2007;56(4):545–52.
41. Saleem N, Patel F, Watkins JL, et al. Timing of ERCP after extracorporeal shock wave lithotripsy for large main pancreatic duct stones. Surg Endosc 2023. https://doi.org/10.1007/s00464-023-10467-2.
42. Brand B, Kahl M, Sidhu S, et al. Prospective evaluation of morphology, function, and quality of life after extracorporeal shockwave lithotripsy and endoscopic treatment of chronic calcific pancreatitis. Am J Gastroenterol 2000;95(12):3428–38.
43. Merrill JT, Mullady DK, Early DS, et al. Timing of endoscopy after extracorporeal shock wave lithotripsy for chronic pancreatitis. Pancreas 2011;40(7):1087–90.
44. Guo JY, Qian YY, Sun H, et al. Optimal Timing of Endoscopic Intervention After Extracorporeal Shock-Wave Lithotripsy in the Treatment of Chronic Calcified Pancreatitis. Pancreas 2021;50(4):633–8.
45. Ohyama H, Mikata R, Ishihara T, et al. Efficacy of stone density on noncontrast computed tomography in predicting the outcome of extracorporeal shock wave lithotripsy for patients with pancreatic stones. Pancreas 2015;44(3):422–8.
46. Adamek HE, Jakobs R, Buttmann A, et al. Long term follow up of patients with chronic pancreatitis and pancreatic stones treated with extracorporeal shock wave lithotripsy. Gut 1999;45:402–5.
47. Choi EK, McHenry L, Watkins JL, et al. Use of intravenous secretin during extracorporeal shock wave lithotripsy to facilitate endoscopic clearance of pancreatic duct stones. Pancreatology 2012;12:272–5.
48. Hu LH, Ye B, Yang YG, et al. Extracorporeal Shock Wave Lithotripsy for Chinese Patients With Pancreatic Stones: A Prospective Study of 214 Cases. Pancreas 2016;45(2):298–305.
49. Korpela T, Udd M, Tenca A, et al. Long-term results of combined ESWL and ERCP treatment of chronic calcific pancreatitis. Scand J Gastroenterol 2016; 51:866–71.
50. Brewer Gutierrez OI, Raijman I, Shah RJ, et al. Safety and efficacy of digital single-operator pancreatoscopy for obstructing pancreatic ductal stones. Endosc Int Open 2019;7(7):E896–903.
51. Beyna T, Neuhaus H, Gerges C. Endoscopic treatment of pancreatic duct stones under direct vision: Revolution or resignation? Systematic review. Dig Endosc 2018;30(1):29–37.
52. Leifsson BG, Borgström A, Ahlgren G. Splenic rupture following ESWL for a pancreatic duct calculus. Dig Surg 2001;18(3):229–30.
53. Udayakumar N, Muhammad KH, Kiran K, et al. Digital, single-operator cholangiopancreatoscopy in the diagnosis and management of pancreatobiliary disorders: a multicenter clinical experience (with video). Gastrointest Endosc 2016; 84(4):649–55.
54. Vassar GJ, Chan KF, Teichman JM, et al. Holmium: YAG lithotripsy: photothermal mechanism. J Endourol 1999;13(3):181–90.
55. De Luca L, Repici A, Kocollari A, et al. Pancreatoscopy: An update. World J Gastrointest Endosc 2019;11(1):22–30.
56. Gerges C, Albers D, Schmitz L, et al. Digital single-operator pancreatoscopy for the treatment of symptomatic pancreatic duct stones: a prospective multicenter cohort trial. Endoscopy 2022;55(02):150–7.

57. Attwell AR, Patel S, Kahaleh M, et al. ERCP with per-oral pancreatoscopy-guided laser lithotripsy for calcific chronic pancreatitis: a multicenter U.S. experience. Gastrointest Endosc 2015;82(2):311–8.
58. Ito K, Igarashi Y, Okano N, et al. Efficacy of combined endoscopic lithotomy and extracorporeal shock wave lithotripsy, and additional electrohydraulic lithotripsy using the SpyGlass direct visualization system or X-ray guided EHL as needed, for pancreatic lithiasis. BioMed Res Int 2014;2014:732781.
59. Ogura T, Okuda A, Imanishi M, et al. Electrohydraulic Lithotripsy for Pancreatic Duct Stones Under Digital Single-Operator Pancreatoscopy (with Video). Dig Dis Sci 2019;64(5):1377–82.
60. Attwell AR, Brauer BC, Chen YK, et al. Endoscopic retrograde cholangiopancreatography with per oral pancreatoscopy for calcific chronic pancreatitis using endoscope and catheter-based pancreatoscopes: a 10-year single-center experience. Pancreas 2014;43(2):268–74.
61. Han S, Shah RJ, Brauer BC, et al. A Comparison of Endoscopic Retrograde Pancreatography With or Without Pancreatoscopy for Removal of Pancreatic Duct Stones. Pancreas 2019;48(5):690–7.
62. Saghir SM, Mashiana HS, Mohan BP, et al. Efficacy of pancreatoscopy for pancreatic duct stones: A systematic review and meta-analysis. World J Gastroenterol 2020;26(34):5207–19.
63. McCarty TR, Sobani Z, Rustagi T. Per-oral pancreatoscopy with intraductal lithotripsy for difficult pancreatic duct stones: a systematic review and meta-analysis. Endosc Int Open 2020;8(10):E1460–70.
64. van der Wiel SE, Stassen PMC, Poley JW, et al. Pancreatoscopy-guided electrohydraulic lithotripsy for the treatment of obstructive pancreatic duct stones: a prospective consecutive case series. Gastrointest Endosc 2022;95(5): 905–914 e2.
65. Seza K, Yamaguchi T, Ishihara T, et al. A long-term controlled trial of endoscopic pancreatic stenting for treatment of main pancreatic duct stricture in chronic pancreatitis. Hepato-Gastroenterology Nov-Dec 2011;58(112):2128–31.
66. Ponchon T, Bory RM, Hedelius F, et al. Endoscopic stenting for pain relief in chronic pancreatitis: results of a standardized protocol. Gastrointest Endosc 1995;42:452–6.
67. Tringali A, Bove V, Vadalà di Prampero SF, et al. Long-term follow-up after multiple plastic stenting for refractory pancreatic duct strictures in chronic pancreatitis. Endoscopy 2019;51(10):930–5.
68. Costamagna G, Bulajic M, Tringali A, et al. Multiple stenting of refractory pancreatic duct strictures in severe chronic pancreatitis: long-term results. Endoscopy 2006;38(3):254–9.
69. Ang TL. Endoscopic management of pancreatic duct stricture in chronic pancreatitis: Are fully covered self-expandable metallic stents ready for prime time? J Gastroenterol Hepatol 2020;35(7):1093–4.
70. Han S, Obando JV, Bhatt A, et al. Biliary and pancreatic stents. Gastrointest Endosc 2023;97(6):1003–4.
71. Boursier J, Quentin V, Le Tallec V, et al. Endoscopic treatment of painful chronic pancreatitis: evaluation of a new flexible multiperforated plastic stent. Gastroenterol Clin Biol 2008;32(10):801–5.
72. Sauer BG, Gurka MJ, Ellen K, et al. Effect of pancreatic duct stent diameter on hospitalization in chronic pancreatitis: does size matter? Pancreas 2009;38: 728–31.

73. Smits ME, Badiga SM, Rauws EA, et al. Long-term results of pancreatic stents in chronic pancreatitis. Gastrointest Endosc 1995;42:461–7.

74. Topazian M, Aslanian H, Andersen D. Outcome following endoscopic stenting of pancreatic duct strictures in chronic pancreatitis. J Clin Gastroenterol 2005;39: 908–11.

75. He YX, Xu HW, Sun XT, et al. Endoscopic management of early-stage chronic pancreatitis based on M-ANNHEIM classification system: a prospective study. Pancreas 2014;43:829–33.

76. Hirota M, Asakura T, Kanno A, et al. Long-period pancreatic stenting for painful chronic calcified pancreatitis required higher medical costs and frequent hospitalizations compared with surgery. Pancreas 2011;40:946–50.

77. Weber A, Schneider J, Neu B, et al. Endoscopic stent therapy in patients with chronic pancreatitis: a 5-year follow-up study. World J Gastroenterol 2013;19: 715–20.

78. Li TT, Song SL, Xiao LN, et al. Efficacy of fully covered self-expandable metal stents for the management of pancreatic duct strictures in chronic pancreatitis: A systematic review and meta-analysis. J Gastroenterol Hepatol 2020;35(7): 1099–106.

79. Lee SH, Kim YS, Kim EJ, et al. Long-term outcomes of fully covered self-expandable metal stents versus plastic stents in chronic pancreatitis. Sci Rep 2021;11(1):15637.

80. Sofi AA, Khan MA, Ahmad S, et al. Comparison of clinical outcomes of multiple plastic stents and covered metal stent in refractory pancreatic ductal strictures in chronic pancreatitis- a systematic review and meta-analysis. Pancreatology 2021;21(5):854–61.

81. Moon SH, Kim MH, Park DH, et al. Modified fully covered self-expandable metal stents with antimigration features for benign pancreatic-duct strictures in advanced chronic pancreatitis, with a focus on the safety profile and reducing migration. Gastrointest Endosc 2010;72(1):86–91.

82. Lee YN, Moon JH, Park JK, et al. Preliminary study of a modified, nonflared, short, fully covered metal stent for refractory benign pancreatic duct strictures (with videos). Gastrointest Endosc 2020;91(4):826–33.

83. Park DH, Kim MH, Moon SH, et al. Feasibility and safety of placement of a newly designed, fully covered self-expandable metal stent for refractory benign pancreatic ductal strictures: a pilot study (with video). Gastrointest Endosc 2008;68(6):1182–9.

84. Ko SW, So H, Oh D, et al. Long-term clinical outcomes of a fully covered self-expandable metal stent for refractory pancreatic strictures in symptomatic chronic pancreatitis: An 11-year follow-up study. J Gastroenterol Hepatol 2023;38(3):460–7.

85. Sherman S, Kozarek RA, Costamagna G, et al. Soft self-expandable metal stent to treat painful pancreatic duct strictures secondary to chronic pancreatitis: a prospective multicenter trial. Gastrointest Endosc 2023;97(3):472–81.e3.

86. Sauer B, Talreja J, Ellen K, et al. Temporary placement of a fully covered self-expandable metal stent in the pancreatic duct for management of symptomatic refractory chronic pancreatitis: preliminary data (with videos). Gastrointest Endosc 2008;68(6):1173–8.

87. Farnbacher MJ, Muhldorfer S, Wehler M, et al. Interventional endoscopic therapy in chronic pancreatitis including temporary stenting: a definitive treatment? Scand J Gastroenterol 2006;41(1):111–7.

88. Bakman YG, Safdar K, Freeman ML. Significant clinical implications of prophylactic pancreatic stent placement in previously normal pancreatic ducts. Endoscopy 2009;41(12):1095–8.
89. Ramchandani M, Pal P, Costamagna G. Management of Benign Biliary Stricture in Chronic Pancreatitis. Gastrointest Endosc Clin N Am 2023;33(4):831–44.
90. Familiari P, Boskoski I, Bove V, et al. ERCP for biliary strictures associated with chronic pancreatitis. Gastrointest Endosc Clin N Am 2013;23(4):833–45.
91. Abdallah AA, Krige JE, Bornman PC. Biliary tract obstruction in chronic pancreatitis. HPB (Oxford) 2007;9(6):421–8.
92. Hao L, Bi Y-W, Zhang D, et al. Risk Factors and Nomogram for Common Bile Duct Stricture in Chronic Pancreatitis: A Cohort of 2153 Patients. J Clin Gastroenterol 2019;53(3):e91–100.
93. Regimbeau JM, Fuks D, Bartoli E, et al. A comparative study of surgery and endoscopy for the treatment of bile duct stricture in patients with chronic pancreatitis. Surg Endosc 2012;26(10):2902–8.
94. Liu Y, Yin XY, Hu LH. Comments on Study of Single Metal Stent and Multiple Plastic Stents Insertion for Benign Biliary Strictures Secondary to Chronic Pancreatitis. Gastroenterology 2022;162(1):346.
95. Catalano MF, Linder JD, George S, et al. Treatment of symptomatic distal common bile duct stenosis secondary to chronic pancreatitis: comparison of single vs. multiple simultaneous stents. Gastrointest Endosc 2004;60(6):945–52.
96. Udd M, Kylänpää L, Kokkola A. The Role of Endoscopic and Surgical Treatment in Chronic Pancreatitis. Scand J Surg 2020;109(1):69–78.
97. Coté GA, Slivka A, Tarnasky P, et al. Effect of Covered Metallic Stents Compared With Plastic Stents on Benign Biliary Stricture Resolution: A Randomized Clinical Trial. JAMA 22-29 2016;315(12):1250–7.
98. Ramchandani M, Lakhtakia S, Costamagna G, et al. Fully Covered Self-Expanding Metal Stent vs Multiple Plastic Stents to Treat Benign Biliary Strictures Secondary to Chronic Pancreatitis: A Multicenter Randomized Trial. Gastroenterology 2021;161(1):185–95.
99. Lakhtakia S, Reddy N, Dolak W, et al. Long-term outcomes after temporary placement of a self-expanding fully covered metal stent for benign biliary strictures secondary to chronic pancreatitis. Gastrointest Endosc 2020;91(2):361–9.
100. Sharaiha RZ, Novikov A, Weaver K, et al. Fully covered self-expanding metal stents for refractory pancreatic duct strictures in symptomatic chronic pancreatitis, US experience. Endosc Int Open 2019;7(11):E1419–23.
101. Papalavrentios L, Musala C, Gkolfakis P, et al. Multiple stents are not superior to single stent insertionfor pain relief in patients with chronic pancreatitis: a retrospective comparative study. Endosc Int Open 2019;7:E1595–604.

Approaches to Pancreaticobiliary Endoscopy in Roux-en-Y Gastric Bypass Anatomy

Khaled Elfert, MD[a], Michel Kahaleh, MD[b],*

KEYWORDS

- Endoscopic retrograde cholangiopancreatography
- EUS-directed transgastric ERCP • Roux-en-Y gastric bypass
- Lumen-apposing metal stent

KEY POINTS

- Performing endoscopic retrograde cholangiopancreatography (ERCP) in Roux-en-Y gastric bypass patients is challenging due to altered anatomy. Various techniques, such as laparoscopy-assisted ERCP (LA-ERCP) and enteroscopy-assisted ERCP, have been used, each with its challenges.
- Endoscopic ultrasound-directed transgastric ERCP (EDGE) creates a fistula between the gastric pouch or jejunum and excluded stomach utilizing a lumen-apposing metal stent (LAMS) placement, allowing ERCP through the LAMS.
- The EDGE indication has been expanded beyond the management of biliary duct pathologies to encompass a wide range of luminal and extraluminal indications.
- EDGE has higher technical success and shorter procedure time than enteroscopy assisted ERCP (E-Ercp). EDGE's technical success rate is equivalent to LA-ERCP. However, EDGE has a lower rate of adverse events, lower costs, and shorter procedure time and hospital stay.
- Common adverse events include perforation, stent migration, bleeding, and fistula persistence, most of which can be managed endoscopically. Persistent fistula rates increase with longer LAMS dwell time.

INTRODUCTION

The rise in obesity rates in recent decades has been associated with an increased prevalence of bariatric surgeries. One of the common bariatric surgeries is Roux-en-Y

[a] SBH Health System, CUNY School of Medicine, 4422 3rd Avenue, Bronx, NY 10457, USA;
[b] Department of Gastroenterology, Robert Wood Johnson University Hospital, RWJ Place, MEB 464, New Brunswick, NJ 08901, USA
* Corresponding author.
E-mail address: mkahaleh@gmail.com

Gastrointest Endoscopy Clin N Am 34 (2024) 475–486
https://doi.org/10.1016/j.giec.2024.02.009
1052-5157/24/© 2024 Elsevier Inc. All rights reserved.

gastric bypass (RYGB). The alteration of normal anatomy in RYGB poses challenges in performing endoscopic retrograde cholangiopancreatography (ERCP) due to the difficulty in reaching the ampulla of Vater endoscopically. To overcome this challenge, different techniques have been proposed to approach the ampulla.

One such technique is to perform laparoscopy to obtain access for ERCP.[1] In this approach the surgeon creates a gastrostomy to the excluded stomach (gastric remnant) to allow a standard duodenoscope to pass to the duodenum. This intraoperative ERCP approach is associated with high technical and clinical success rates but is also linked to longer hospital stays and procedure time.[2]

Another modality is enteroscopy-assisted ERCP, which utilizes enteroscopy to reach the ampulla retrograde through the afferent (biliopancreatic limb).[3] This procedure has a lower rate of severe adverse events compared to laparoscopy-assisted ERCP (LA-ERCP) but with suboptimal technical and clinical success rates. This is due to the acute angulations and a long afferent limb, leading to difficulty in reaching the ampulla to perform ERCP.[4,5] In addition to the technical difficulties in reaching the papilla, the use of a forward-viewing endoscope and the relative lack of accessories are disadvantages.

Recently, a new procedure has emerged that utilizes a lumen-apposing metal stent (LAMS) to create a fistula between the stomach pouch or jejunum and the gastric remnant, allowing the performance of traditional ERCP through the excluded stomach. This procedure also facilitates the performance of diagnostic and therapeutic endoscopic ultrasound (EUS) through the LAMS, procedures that were previously very difficult to perform in patients with RYGB.[6]

Technique

Overall review of the procedure technique

After examination of the stomach and afferent limb using diagnostic endoscopy, a linear echoendoscope is advanced into the stomach pouch. The gastric remnant is visualized endosonographically (**Fig. 1**). Afterward, a 19 G needle is advanced from the gastric pouch or the afferent limb into the excluded stomach. Contrast mixed with water is injected to distend the stomach and visualize it fluoroscopically (**Fig. 2**). The needle can be attached to a standard waterjet system to allow distension. A cautery-enhanced LAMS is used to create the fistula. The distal flange is deployed first into the excluded stomach under fluoroscopic and endosonographic guidance (**Fig. 3**). The proximal flange is then deployed into the stomach pouch or the afferent jejunal loop (**Fig. 4**). This is followed by the dilation of the stent to the diameter of the stent using a dilating balloon (**Fig. 5**), if a single-stage EDGE and ERCP are performed. Once the fistulized tract is created, a duodenoscope or echoendoscope is advanced

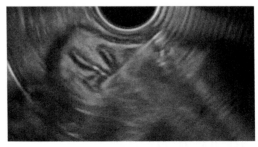

Fig. 1. Visualization of the excluded stomach by endosonography and puncture with a 19 G needle.

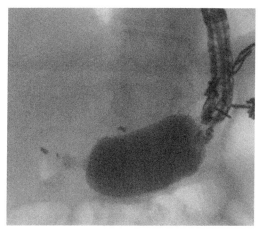

Fig. 2. Filling of the excluded stomach with a mixture of contrast and water under fluoroscopy.

through the LAMS to perform ERCP or EUS (**Fig. 6**). This can be performed at the index procedure or a subsequent procedure. After completion of the ERCP, the LAMS is removed, the timing of which is related to tract maturation, which occurs at 3 to 4 weeks. The resultant fistula is either left to close spontaneously or closed endoscopically using an over-the-scope clip or endoscopic suturing.

One-stage versus two-stage endoscopic ultrasound-directed transgastric endoscopic retrograde cholangiopancreatography

ERCP is usually performed in a subsequent session following EDGE to allow for maturation of the tract, since stent dislodgement during passage of the ERCP scope at the initial session results in perforation. A single-stage EDGE is performed when the indication for ERCP is urgent, such as in the management of cholangitis. **Table 1** demonstrates the proportion of procedures performed as single stage and as two stages in different studies.

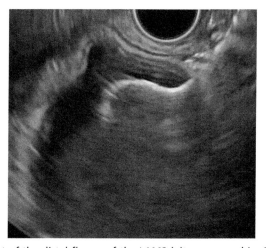

Fig. 3. Deployment of the distal flange of the LAMS (ultrasonographic view).

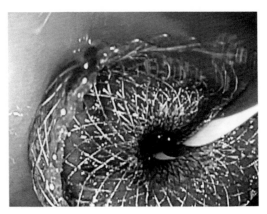

Fig. 4. Deployment of the proximal flange of the LAMS (endoscopic view).

Access for endoscopic ultrasound-directed transgastric endoscopic retrograde cholangiopancreatography

The initial EDGE access is usually done through the stomach remnant or through the proximal part of the afferent jejunal loop (**Table 2**). Multiple factors determine the selection of the access point, including the presence of intervening vessels, the proximity of the access location to the excluded stomach, the intent of deploying the distal flange of the LAMS in the gastric body or gastric antrum, and the patient's anatomy.

Removal of Lumen-apposing metal stent

LAMS removal occurs once the need for access is no longer required and after the tract has matured. In a small percentage of cases, there is a persistent fistula at the site of LAMS. Options for managing a persistent fistula range from no intervention to active endoscopic treatments. These treatments may include argon plasma coagulation of the tract edges to encourage healing or closing the endoscopic edges using devices like endoscopic suturing, over-the-scope clipping, or traditional through-the-scope clipping. The method chosen often hinges on the endoscopist's preference, and currently, no studies compare the efficacy of these various fistula-closing approaches.[11,14] If the fistula cannot be closed endoscopically and the patient experiences significant weight gain, or marginal ulceration that can be complicated by

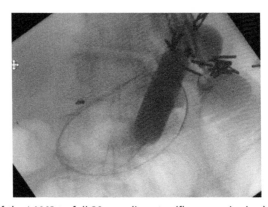

Fig. 5. Dilation of the LAMS to full 20 mm diameter (fluoroscopic view).

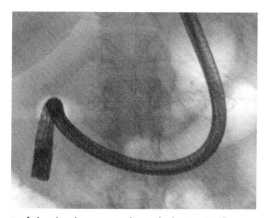

Fig. 6. Advancement of the duodenoscope through the LAMS (fluoroscopic view).

persistent epigastric pain and risk of upper gastrointestinal bleeding, then surgical repair is indicated.

Stent type. The most commonly used stent type is LAMS (AXIOS, Boston Scientific, Marlborough, MA). However, in a study by de Benito and colleagues, 4 of 14 procedures were performed using large-diameter self-expandable metal stents.[10] LAMS are typically preferred since they have a well-documented appositional force and are easily deployed because of the electrocautery-enhanced tip.[20]

Stent size

Different options for LAMS stent sizes include 15 and 20 mm. The choice is based on endoscopic preference, availability, and saddle length as the 15 mm diameter is also available in 15 mm length compared to the 20 mm that has a length of 10 mm. The larger diameter is seemingly linked to a higher technical success rate. A multicenter

Table 1		
Single-stage vs two-stage endoscopic ultrasound-directed transgastric ERCP across different studies		
Study, Year, Country	**Single Stage**	**Two Stages**
James et al,[7] 2019[a] USA	14/19 (73.68%)	4/19 (21.05%)
Kedia et al,[8] 2019 [c] USA	0/29 (0%)	29/29 (100%)
Krafft et al,[9] 2019[c] USA	5/14 (35.71%)	9/14 (64.29%)
De Benito SM,[10] 2020[a] Spain	10/10 (100%)	0/10 (0%)
Runge et al,[11] 2021[c] USA & UK	88/175 (50.29%)	87/175 (49.71%)
Tyberg et al,[12] 2020[a] USA	5/19 (26.32%)	14/19 (73.68%)
Shinn et al,[13] 2021 USA[c]	128/128 (100%)	0/128 (0%)
Bahdi et al,[14] 2022[a] USA	17/32 (53.12%)	15/32 (46.88%)
Ghandour et al,[15] 2022 USA and UK[c]	17/47 (36.2%)	30/47 (63.8%)
Chhabra et al,[16] 2022 UK[b]	8/14 (57.1%)	6/14 (42.9%)
Krafft et al,[17] 2022 USA[b]	9/22 (41%)	13/22 (59%)

[a] Single-center study.
[b] Dual-center Study.
[c] Multicenter study.

Table 2
Access routes in endoscopic ultrasound-directed transgastric ERCP procedure

Study, Year, Country	Gastro-Gastric Fistula	Jejunogastric Fistula
Full		
James et al,[7] 2019[a] USA	8/19 (42.11%)	11/19 (57.89%)
Krafft et al,[9] 2019[c] USA	8/14 (57.14%)	6/14 (42.86%)
De Benito SM,[10] 2020 USA[a]	5/10 (50.00%)	5/10 (50.00%)
Kochhar et al,[18] 2020 USA[a]	22/26 (84.62%)	4/26 (15.38%)
Runge et al,[11] 2021 USA and UK,[c]	88/175 (50.29%)	87/175 (49.71%)
Tyberg et al,[12] 2020 USA[a]	17/19 (89.47%)	2/19 (10.53%)
Shinn et al,[13] 2021 USA[c]	89/128 (69.53%)	39/128 (30.47%)
Bahdi et al,[14] 2022 USA[a]	23/32 (71.88%)	9/32 (28.13%)
Ghandour et al,[15] 2022 USA and UK[c]	37/47 (78.87%)	10/47 (21.3%)
Chhabra et al,[16] 2022 UK[b]	11/14 (78.6%)	3/14 (21.4%)
Krafft et al,[17] 2022 USA[b]	12/22 (55%)	10/22 (45%)
Kedia et al,[19] 2023 USA and Spain[c]	125/172 (73%)	47/172 (27%)

[a] Single-center study.
[b] Dual-center Study.
[c] Multicenter study.

retrospective study demonstrated that the 15 mm diameter was associated with higher odds of stent dislodgement in patients undergoing single-session EDGE (OR 5.36; CI 1.29–22.24).[13] Another retrospective study by Bahdi and colleagues found that the 20 mm diameter is associated with a lower rate of adverse events, further supporting its superiority.[14] It is noteworthy that while the 15 mm diameter was more prevalent in the early years of EDGE, the larger diameter has gained traction in recent years, yielding better outcomes (**Table 3**).[19]

Adverse Events and Their Management

Perforation
Perforation is a noted adverse event of the EDGE procedure. The incidence of perforation varied across the studies.[2] Perforation with associated LAMS migration can occur intraprocedurally or postprocedurally.[14] Perforation can happen during initial stent deployment or when stent dislodgement occurs after advancement of the duodenoscope through the stent.[12] Perforation appears to occur more frequently after jejunogastric LAMS placement as compared to gastrogastric LAMS placement.[11] Perforation management depends on the severity and can include laparoscopic closure, endoscopic closure, and conservative treatment.[11] Any risk of peritoneal spillage should dictate closure to prevent increased chance of morbidity.

Stent migration/dislodgement
Stent migration is among the prevalent adverse events of EDGE procedure with reported rates ranging between 15% and 33%.[21–23] Stent migration (dislodgement) can occur either during or after the ERCP procedure. Intraprocedural dislodgement is particularly noticeable in the single-session EDGE and results in perforation. Performing EDGE in two steps decreases the possibility of stent dislodgement and perforation as it allows time for fistula maturation and stabilization of the LAMS. Techniques that may mitigate the likelihood of EDGE stent dislodgement include stent suturing, stent dilation, and the use of larger diameter stent. Shinn and colleagues demonstrated

Table 3
The size of the lumen apposing metal stent used in endoscopic ultrasound-directed transgastric ERCP studies

Study, Year, Country	15 mm Diameter	20 mm Diameter
Tyberg et al,[21] 2017 USA[b]	16/16	0/16
Bukhari et al,[3] 2018 USA and Denmark[c]	30/30	0/30
Kedia et al,[8] 2019 USA[c]	29/29	0/29
Krafft et al,[9] 2019 USA[c]	6/14	8/14
James et al,[7] 2019 USA[a]	19/19	0/19
Kochhar et al,[18] 2020 USA[a]	24/26	2/26
Tyberg et al,[12] 2020 USA[a]	19/19	0/19
Runge et al,[11] 2021 USA and UK[c]	112/178	66/178
Shinn et al,[13] 2021 USA[c]	43/128	85/128
Bahdi et al,[14] 2022 USA[a]	14/32	17/32
Chhabra et al,[16] 2022 UK[b]	0/20	20/20
Ghandour et al,[15] 2022 USA and UK[c]	21/47	26/47
Krafft et al,[17] 2022 USA[b]	0/22	22/22
Kedia et al,[19] 2023 USA and Spain[c]	32/172	140/172

[a] Single-center study.
[b] Dual-center Study.
[c] Multicenter study.

that the only factor associated with a higher likelihood of stent dislodgement during single-stage EDGE with ERCP is smaller stent size (stent size 15 vs 20 mm, OR 5.271, CI 1.47–18.86, P 0.007).[13] A recent multicenter study by Kedia and colleagues analyzed the association between various technical factors and stent migration/ dislodgement. Their findings indicated a trend toward a higher migration rate with smaller stent diameter and single-session procedure; however, the differences were not statistically significant.[19] Intraprocedural stent dislodgement can usually be managed by placement of bridging stents including overlapping LAMS or TTS esophageal stents. When successful, surgical intervention is rarely needed, postprocedural stent migration can be managed by repositioning/replacing the stent or allowing it to pass enterally.[19]

Bleeding
Bleeding can occur at various times during the procedure. It can occur during fistula creation or because of the sphincterotomy performed during ERCP. Bleeding from the fistula site can be controlled using bridging stent placement for tamponade.[10]

Fistula persistence
One of the sequelae of the EDGE procedure is the persistence of the gastrogastric/jejunogastric fistula. After LAMS removal, the decision between actively closing the fistula and allowing it to close spontaneously is usually left to endoscopist's preference. The only factor that was associated with a higher rate of fistula persistence was a longer LAMS dwell time. Krafft and colleagues showed that in patients in whom the fistula was left to heal by secondary intent, patients with persistent fistula had longer LAMS dwell time compared to patients with durable fistula closure (median of 77 days vs 35 days, P 0.03).[17] These findings were confirmed by Kedia and colleagues in their multicenter study that included patients who had active 49% (69 of 142) and spontaneous

fistula closure 51% (73 of 142). The median LAMS dwell time in the persistent fistula group was 86 days as opposed to 50 days in the patients without persistent fistula group (P 0.004). Interestingly, in patients who underwent evaluation for fistula persistence, there was no discernible difference in the rates of fistula persistence between patients who had undergone active fistula closure and those who had not.[19]

Weight gain

Post-EDGE weight gain can arise due to the persistence of the fistula between gastric pouch or jejunum and the excluded stomach. In a recent meta-analysis conducted by Deliwala and colleagues, the pooled rate of post-EDGE weight gain was 4% (2–9, $I^2 = 0\%$), and the mean weight change across all the studies included in the meta-analysis was −0.53 lbs.[2] Notably, the median weight change was actually negative in multiple retrospective studies.[11,14] In a study encompassing 172 patients, weight gain was noted in 63 patients while LAMS was in place. Out of those patients who gained weight, 59% (38 of 63) gained less than 5 lbs.[19]

Endoscopic ultrasound-directed transgastric intervention

EUS-directed transgastric intervention (EDGI) refers to the use of the same technique of EDGE procedure to access the excluded stomach to perform endoscopic procedures other than ERCP.[9,15] The indications for EDGI fall into 2 main categories. The first category includes accessing the excluded stomach for luminal indications, for example, gastroduodenal luminal biopsy for mass lesions and therapeutic procedures for gastric or duodenal ulcers. The other category includes the evaluation and the treatment of extraluminal pathologies near the excluded stomach and the duodenum utilizing EUS, for example, EUS-guided FNB of suspected cholangiocarcinoma and drainage of pancreatic fluid collection. This broadened scope of the technique highlights the procedure's versatility, making it a valuable tool in both luminal and extraluminal endoscopic interventions.[9]

Comparison to Other Procedures

EDGE is an effective procedure with a pooled technical success rate and clinical success rate of 96% and 91%, according to a recently published meta-analysis.[2]

E-endoscopic retrograde cholangiopancreatography

Device-assisted endoscopic procedures that can be used to assist the performance of ERCP include double-balloon enteroscopy, single-balloon endoscopy, and spiral enteroscopy. Double- and single-balloon enteroscopies were initially developed for deep exploration of the small bowel in 2001 and later utilized for reaching out to the papilla to perform ERCP in patients with RYGB.[24,25]

Spiral enteroscopy is another modality that was developed as an alternative to balloon-assisted enteroscopy and has been used to facilitate ERCP in patients with altered anatomy.[26] A multicenter US study demonstrated that the ERCP success rate in patients who undergo enteroscopy-assisted ERCP is 63% with no statistically significant difference in enteroscopy success rate between different methods.[27]

It is important to note that enteroscopy-assisted ERCP is only an option for biliary indications and is generally not useful for pancreatic indications.

Endoscopic ultrasound-directed transgastric endoscopic retrograde cholangiopancreatography versus enteroscopy-assisted endoscopic retrograde cholangiopancreatography

Compared to enteroscopy-associated ERCP, EDGE is superior in terms of technical success rate. It also results in shorter procedure time (61 vs 169 minutes, P 0.04) and shorter hospital stay (1.8 vs 6.9 days, $P < .001$). The pooled adverse events rate was lower with EDGE, but the difference was not statistically significant (9.6% vs 16%, P 0.22).[2]

The suboptimal technical success rate of E-ERCP is attributed to different factors including the long afferent limb and the acute angulations due to adhesions making it difficult to reach out to the papilla. Other limitations are the forward-viewing nature of the endoscope and the fact that the working channel is small with a long diameter making it difficult for standard accessories to be used.[28]

Laparoscopy-assisted endoscopic retrograde cholangiopancreatography
LA-ERCP included using laparoscope to create percutaneous access to the excluded stomach followed by insertion of a side-viewing duodenoscopy through the trocar to perform the ERCP procedure.[1]

Endoscopic ultrasound-directed transgastric endoscopic retrograde cholangiopancreatography versus laparoscopy-assisted endoscopic retrograde cholangiopancreatography
EDGE has been shown to have an equivalent technical success rate (97% vs 98%). The adverse event rate was numerically lower in the EDGE group (13 vs 17.6%, P 0.52). Similar to EDGE versus E-ERCP, EDGE was associated with shorter procedure time (75 vs 187 minutes, $P<.001$) and shorter hospital stay (2.5 vs 5.4 days, $P<.001$) compared to LA-ERCP.[2] Moreover, a cost-effectiveness analysis showed that EDGE was superior to E-ERCP and LA-ERCP. It was associated with the lowest total costs, and highest total quality-adjusted life years compared to the other two alternative modalities.[29]

It is worth noting that the higher cost associated with LA-ERCP is related to the utilization of the operating room. In addition, the procedure poses challenges due to the need for coordination between the surgical and the endoscopic teams, which leads to the prolongation of the procedure time. Additionally, the surgical steps required for the procedure contribute to a significant proportion of adverse events.[1]

SUMMARY

EDGE procedure stands out as an established procedure that is used for a wide range of pancreaticobiliary indications in patients with altered anatomy due to RYGB. It offers favorable outcomes and potential benefits over more traditional approaches, for example, E-ERCP and LA-ERCP. Further research and refinement in addressing adverse events are essential to enhance its safety and efficacy, solidifying its position as a valuable tool to facilitate ERCP and EUS in patients with RYGB.

CLINICS CARE POINTS

- Consider EDGE for RYGB patients needing ERCP/EUS, given its favorable outcomes and lower adverse event rates with expertise.

- The LAMS stent is the preferred stent for performing LAMS procedures, attributed to its electrocautery-enhanced tip that facilitates stent placement.

- For nonurgent ERCP cases, it is advisable to opt for a 2 staged EDGE procedure. This approach supports fistula maturation, minimizing the risk of stent dislodgement.

- The choice between gastrogastric and jejunogastric access for EDGE depends on various factors, including patient anatomy and the intended deployment of the distal flange.

- LAMS dwell time predicts fistula persistence after LAMS removal, and the smaller stent size is associated with higher rate of stent dislodgement.
- Addressing persistent fistulas post-LAMS removal may involve allowing them to heal through secondary intention, with potential consideration for endoscopic closure as needed.

DISCLOSURE

K. Elfert has no conflict of interest to disclose. M. Kahaleh has received grant support from Boston Scientific, Fujinon, Apollo Endosurgery, Cook Endoscopy, Olympus, and MI Tech. He is a consultant for Boston Scientific, ABBvie. None of those fundings were related to this study.

REFERENCES

1. Banerjee N, Parepally M, Byrne TK, et al. Systematic review of transgastric ERCP in Roux-en-Y gastric bypass patients. Surg Obes Relat Dis 2017;13(7): 1236–42.
2. Deliwala SS, Mohan BP, Yarra P, et al. Efficacy & safety of EUS-directed transgastric endoscopic retrograde cholangiopancreatography (EDGE) in Roux-en-Y gastric bypass anatomy: a systematic review & meta-analysis. Surg Endosc 2023;37(6):4144–58.
3. Bukhari M, Kowalski T, Nieto J, et al. An international, multicenter, comparative trial of EUS-guided gastrogastrostomy-assisted ERCP versus enteroscopy-assisted ERCP in patients with Roux-en-Y gastric bypass anatomy. Gastrointest Endosc 2018;88(3):486–94.
4. Krutsri C, Kida M, Yamauchi H, et al. Current status of endoscopic retrograde cholangiopancreatography in patients with surgically altered anatomy. World J Gastroenterol 2019;25(26):3313–33.
5. Elfert K, Zeid E, Duarte-Chavez R, et al. Endoscopic ultrasound guided access procedures following surgery. Best Pract Res Clin Gastroenterol 2022;60-61: 101812.
6. Kedia P, Sharaiha RZ, Kumta NA, et al. Internal EUS-directed transgastric ERCP (EDGE): game over. Gastroenterology 2014;147(3):566–8.
7. James TW, Baron TH. Endoscopic ultrasound-directed transgastric ERCP (EDGE): a single-center us experience with follow-up data on fistula closure. Obes Surg 2019;29(2):451–6.
8. Kedia P, Tarnasky PR, Nieto J, et al. EUS-directed transgastric ERCP (EDGE) versus laparoscopy-assisted ERCP (LA-ERCP) for roux-en-y gastric bypass (RYGB) anatomy. J Clin Gastroenterol 2019;53(4):304–8.
9. Krafft MR, Hsueh W, James TW, et al. The EDGI new take on EDGE: EUS-directed transgastric intervention (EDGI), other than ERCP, for Roux-en-Y gastric bypass anatomy: a multicenter study. Endosc Int Open 2019;07(10):E1231–40.
10. de Benito SM, Carbajo AY, Sánchez-Ocaña Hernández R, et al. Endoscopic ultrasound-directed transgastric ERCP in patients with Roux-en-Y gastric bypass using lumen-apposing metal stents or duodenal self-expandable metal stents. A European single-center experience. Rev Esp Enferm Dig 2020;112(3): 211–5.
11. Runge TM, Chiang AL, Kowalski TE, et al. Endoscopic ultrasound-directed transgastric ERCP (EDGE): a retrospective multicenter study. Endoscopy 2021;53(06): 611–8.

12. Tyberg A, Kedia P, Tawadros A, et al. EUS-Directed Transgastric Endoscopic Retrograde Cholangiopancreatography (EDGE). J Clin Gastroenterol 2020;54(6): 569–72.
13. Shinn B, Boortalary T, Raijman I, et al. Maximizing success in single-session EUS-directed transgastric ERCP: a retrospective cohort study to identify predictive factors of stent migration. Gastrointest Endosc 2021;94(4):727–32.
14. Bahdi F, George R, Paneerselvam K, et al. Comparison of endoscopic ultrasound-directed transgastric endoscopic retrograde cholangiopancreatography outcomes using various technical approaches. Endosc Int Open 2022;10(04): E459–67.
15. Ghandour B, Shinn B, Dawod QM, et al. EUS-directed transgastric interventions in Roux-en-Y gastric bypass anatomy: a multicenter experience. Gastrointest Endosc 2022;96(4):630–8.
16. Chhabra P, On W, Paranandi B, et al. Initial United Kingdom experience of endoscopic ultrasound-directed transgastric endoscopic retrograde cholangiopancreatography. Ann Hepatobiliary Pancreat Surg 2022;26(4):318–24.
17. Krafft MR, Lorenze A, Croglio MP, et al. "Innocent as a LAMS": Does Spontaneous Fistula Closure (Secondary Intention), After EUS-Directed Transgastric ERCP (EDGE) via 20-mm Lumen-Apposing Metal Stent, Confer an Increased Risk of Persistent Fistula and Unintentional Weight Gain? Dig Dis Sci 2022;67(6):2337.
18. Kochhar GS, Mohy-ud-din N, Grover A, et al. EUS-directed transgastric endoscopic retrograde cholangiopancreatography versus laparoscopic-assisted ERCP versus deep enteroscopy-assisted ERCP for patients with RYGB. Endosc Int Open 2020;8(7):E877–82.
19. Kedia P, Shah-Khan S, Tyberg A, et al. Endoscopic ultrasound-directed transgastric ERCP (EDGE): A multicenter US study on long-term follow-up and fistula closure. Endosc Int Open 2023;11(05):E529–37.
20. Teoh AY, Ng EK, Chan SM, et al. Ex vivo comparison of the lumen-apposing properties of EUS-specific stents (with video). Gastrointest Endosc 2016;84(1):62–8.
21. Tyberg A, Nieto J, Salgado S, et al. Endoscopic Ultrasound (EUS)-Directed Transgastric Endoscopic Retrograde Cholangiopancreatography or EUS: Mid-Term Analysis of an Emerging Procedure. Clin Endosc 2017;50(2):185–90.
22. Ngamruengphong S Nieto JKR, Nieto J, Kunda R, et al. Endoscopic ultrasound-guided creation of a transgastric fistula for the management of hepatobiliary disease in patients with Roux-en-Y gastric bypass. Endoscopy 2017;49(6):549–52.
23. Wang TJ, Cortes P, Jirapinyo P, et al. A comparison of clinical outcomes and cost utility among laparoscopy, enteroscopy, and temporary gastric access-assisted ERCP in patients with Roux-en-Y gastric bypass anatomy. Surg Endosc 2020; 35(8):4469–77.
24. Yamamoto H, Sekine Y, Sato Y, et al. Total enteroscopy with a nonsurgical steerable double-balloon method. Gastrointest Endosc 2001;53(2):216–20.
25. Aabakken L, Bretthauer M, Line PD. Double-balloon enteroscopy for endoscopic retrograde cholangiography in patients with a Roux-en-Y anastomosis. Endoscopy 2007;39(12):1068–71.
26. Ali MF, Modayil R, Gurram KC, et al. Spiral enteroscopy-assisted ERCP in bariatric-length Roux-en-Y anatomy: a large single-center series and review of the literature (with video). Gastrointest Endosc 2018;87(5):1241–7.
27. Shah RJ, Smolkin M, Yen R, et al. A multicenter, U.S. experience of single-balloon, double-balloon, and rotational overtube–assisted enteroscopy ERCP in patients with surgically altered pancreaticobiliary anatomy (with video). Gastrointest Endosc 2013;77(4):593–600.

28. Khara HS, Parvataneni S, Park S, et al. Review of ERCP Techniques in Roux-en-Y Gastric Bypass Patients: Highlight on the Novel EUS-Directed Transgastric ERCP (EGDE) Technique. Curr Gastroenterol Rep 2021;23(7):10.
29. James HJ, James TW, Wheeler SB, et al. Cost-effectiveness of endoscopic ultrasound-directed transgastric ERCP compared with device-assisted and laparoscopic-assisted ERCP in patients with Roux-en-Y anatomy. Endoscopy 2019;51(11):1051–8.

Endoscopic Ultrasound-Guided Biliary Drainage (EUS-BD)

Andrew Canakis, DO[a], Amy Tyberg, MD[b],*

KEYWORDS

- ERCP • Transhepatic biliary drainage • Hepaticogastrostomy
- Choledochoduodenostomy • Lumen-apposing metal stent

KEY POINTS

- Endoscopic ultrasound-guided biliary drainage (EUS-BD) has become an acceptable alternative therapy for biliary decompression when conventional endoscopic retrograde cholangiopancreatography (ERCP) is unsuccessful with improved outcomes compared to percutaneous transhepatic biliary drainage.
- In malignant biliary obstruction, EUS-BD is proven non-inferior and possibly superior to conventional ERCP.
- EUS-BD can be performed via an intrahepatic or extrahepatic approach, and stenting can be performed via a rendezvous approach, antegrade placement, or transluminal placement via hepaticogastrostomy or choledochoduodenostomy. No consensus exists on which technique is superior and approach should be individualized.
- Procedural complexity and lack of dedicated procedural equipment have been limiting factors to the widespread application of these techniques.
- EUS-BD prior to surgical resection seems efficacious and safe; further confirmatory studies are needed.

INTRODUCTION

Endoscopic retrograde cholangiopancreatography (ERCP) with transpapillary stenting is the first-line approach for providing adequate decompression and symptomatic relief for the relief of biliary obstruction. However, unsuccessful cannulation via ERCP occurs in 5% to 10% of cases.[1,2] Factors associated with difficult biliary cannulation include surgically altered anatomy (SAA), periampullary diverticulum, large tumor involvement, and duodenal obstruction.[3] Repeated cannulation attempts (>5 times)

[a] Division of Gastroenterology & Hepatology, University of Maryland School of Medicine, 22 South Greene Street, Baltimore, MD 21201, USA; [b] Hackensack University Medical Center, Hackensack, NJ, USA
* Corresponding author. 186 Rochelle Avenue, Rochelle Park, NJ 07662.
E-mail address: amy.tyberg@gmail.com

Gastrointest Endoscopy Clin N Am 34 (2024) 487–500
https://doi.org/10.1016/j.giec.2023.12.002
1052-5157/24/© 2024 Elsevier Inc. All rights reserved.

and duration (>5 minutes) are also independent predictors of post ERCP pancreatitis.[4] Traditionally, a salvage route of decompression was achieved through percutaneous transhepatic biliary drainage (PTBD) when ERCP failed or was unsuccessful. However, PTBD is associated with substantial rates of morbidity and re-intervention, and tumor seeding in cases of malignancy.[5–7] A large national database study comparing ERCP (n = 7445) and PTBD (n = 1690) showed that endoscopic drainage was associated with lower adverse events (AEs) (8.6% vs 12.3%), shorter hospitalizations (7.6 vs 10.4 days), and lower total costs ($53,881 vs $73,151).[6] Furthermore, the presence of an external catheter may impact the individual's quality of life due to discomfort, cosmetic problems, skin inflammation, dislodgement, and/or bile leakage.[8]

Endoscopic ultrasound-guided biliary drainage (EUS-BD) has emerged as a minimally invasive alternative for biliary drainage when conventional ERCP is not feasible or successful. EUS-BD was first described in 2001 when drainage of the common bile duct was achieved with a transduodenal stent.[9] Since then, EUS-BD has rapidly expanded with advancements in both technique and procedure-related equipment. Indications for EUS-BD have also expanded from purely a rescue therapy after failed ERCP to a first-line approach in cases of SAA or distal obstruction which preclude ERCP access and/or cannulation, and is in some cases utilized as first-line therapy over conventional ERCP in malignant biliary obstruction. Biliary access in EUS-BD can be achieved via an intrahepatic approach through the liver or an extrahepatic approach through the small bowel; stenting can be performed using a rendezvous approach (EUS-RV), antegrade placement, or transluminal (intra or extra hepatic) placement. Transmural intrahepatic stent placement is known as hepaticogastrostomy (HGS); transmural extrahepatic stent placement is known as choledochoduodenostomy (CDS). The optimal drainage strategy depends on the location and etiology of the obstruction. A few contraindications to note are gastric wall tumor infiltration, large volume ascites, severe coagulopathy, an inability to visualize the biliary tract, and presence of intervening vessels.[10]

ENDOSCOPIC ULTRASOUND-GUIDED RENDEZVOUS APPROACH

In patients with intact gastroduodenal anatomy, EUS-RV can be utilized after unsuccessful ERCP cannulation. This technique was first described in a 2004 case series.[11] With this approach, the bile duct is accessed under endoscopic ultrasound (EUS) guidance, and a guidewire is advanced through the biliary tree in antegrade fashion toward the papilla (**Fig. 1**). Puncture routes can be achieved through a transgastric (intrahepatic duct) or transduodenal (extrahepatic duct) from the first or second portion of the duodenum. Some clinicians prefer the intrahepatic method as this may reduce bile leakage thanks to the tamponade effect of surrounding liver parenchyma.[12] Guidewire manipulation is often a challenging step with this technique. Once transpapillary wire access is achieved, the duodenoscope is reinserted. Biliary cannulation is attempted over the EUS-placed guidewire, or the guidewire is grasped and pulled through the working channel of the duodenoscope after which conventional ERCP can be performed.

A recent meta-analysis involving 19 studies with 524 patients found that the overall technical success and AE rate of EUS-RV was 88.7% and 9.8%, respectively.[13] In another study, technical success and AEs between an intra-hepatic versus extra-hepatic approach were not significantly different (65%, 17% vs 87%, 9.8% respectively).[14] Puncture route selection should be individualized based on each patient's anatomy and underlying pathology to ensure technical success, especially since difficult guidewire manipulation is associated with EUS-RV failure. In general, direct EUS-BD

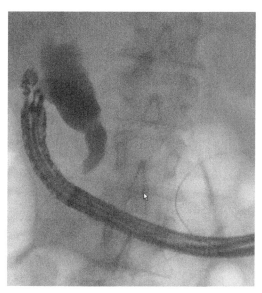

Fig. 1. Fluoroscopic view of an EUS-Guided Rendezvous Approach where a guidewire is advanced through the biliary tree in antegrade fashion towards the papilla.

techniques are more effective than EUS-RV in terms of success rate and procedure time, especially for malignant cases.[15] This technique may be better suited for cases of benign biliary disease.

ENDOSCOPIC ULTRASOUND-GUIDED ANTEGRADE STENTING

In EUS-guided antegrade stenting, the left intrahepatic biliary system is visualized and accessed under EUS via a transgastric puncture. A guidewire is then passed through the biliary tree and across the ampulla or anastomosis into the small bowel. A fistula is created using a dilating balloon with or without cautery, and a stent is advanced antegrade through the biliary tree and deployed across the ampulla or anastomosis. In cases of technical failure, antegrade stenting can be converted to transmural stenting or PTBD.[16] Data using this technique are limited, though studies have reported a pooled technical success rate of 77% and AE rate of 5%.[17–22]

ENDOSCOPIC ULTRASOUND-GUIDED -GUIDED TRANSMURAL STENTING
Endoscopic Ultrasound-Guided Hepaticogastrostomy

EUS-guided hepaticogastrostomy (HGS) involves tract formation between the gastric wall (cardia or lesser curvature) and the left intrahepatic duct (some authors prefer segment III for the puncture site).[10] In this approach, the intrahepatic bile duct is accessed and punctured under EUS visualization and wire access is obtained. A fistula tract is then created using dilation with or without cautery, after which a stent is deployed with the proximal end within the intrahepatic duct and the distal end in the gastric lumen (**Fig. 2**). Technical success of this technique is dependent on sufficient intrahepatic biliary dilation. In addition, other sites of transhepatic drainage such as the esophagus, duodenum, or jejunum (in surgically altered anatomy) have been used as sites. This has led some authors to propose the general term "EUS-guided transhepatic biliary drainage (EUS-TBD)" to mirror PTBD (MOVE REFERENCE 33 AND RENUMBER).

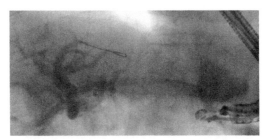

Fig. 2. Fluoroscopic view of an EUS-guided hepaticogastrostomy where a fistula tract is created and a stent is deployed with the proximal end within the intrahepatic duct and the distal end in the gastric lumen.

Endoscopic Ultrasound–Guided Choledochoduodenostomy

EUS-guided choledochoduodenostomy (CDS) is another transluminal technique where a fistula tract is created between the duodenum and extrahepatic bile duct. The extrahepatic bile duct is visualized and accessed using EUS, a guidewire is advanced into the biliary tree and a fistula tract is created with or without cautery (**Fig. 3**). A stent is then deployed with the proximal end in the extrahepatic bile duct and the distal end in the small bowel lumen. In EUS-CDS, the advent of an electrocautery-enhanced lumen-apposing metal stent (LAMS) has allowed for a single step puncture and stent placement (**Figs. 4** and **5**).

Choledochoduodenostomy Versus Hepaticogastrostomy

Choosing between CDS and HGS is based on a multitude of factors related to the location of the obstruction within the biliary tree, the gastroduodenal anatomy, the degree of intrahepatic ductal dilation, and operator preference and experience. In general, HGS is suitable when CDS is not feasible due to SAA, gastric outlet obstruction, or hilar obstruction. Comparative studies have been reported,[23–29] though neither approach is proven superior over the other. Two randomized controlled trials have reported similar rates of technical and clinical success.[25,30] A meta-analysis of 18

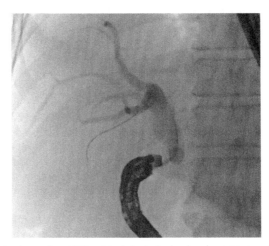

Fig. 3. Fluoroscopic view of an EUS-guided choledochoduodenostomy where a fistula tract is created between the duodenum and extrahepatic bile duct.

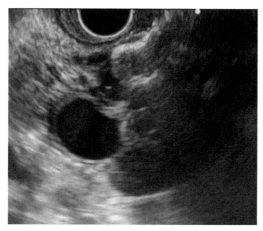

Fig. 4. Endoscopic ultrasound view of an electrocautery-enhanced lumen-apposing metal stent placement for a choledochoduodenostomy.

studies comparing 503 HGS and 473 CDS procedures found that both techniques were similar in terms of technical success, clinical success, and AEs.[31] However, the procedure time and rate of recurrent biliary obstruction was higher for EUS-HGS.

HGS may be preferred over CDS due to a lower risk of a bile leak due to the adjacent liver parenchyma.[32] Similarly, stent misdeployment and/or bleeding in the duodenum or retroperitoneal space may be more difficult to treat compared to the intraperitoneal location.[33] However, some studies suggest HGS may also be associated with higher AEs, which may influence the learning curve and operator preference when choosing between the 2 procedures.[34] Other studies suggest that CDS may be associated with longer stent patency, but possibly higher AEs. A novel algorithm utilized in a single-center study of 52 patients who failed conventional ERCP suggests that deciding on a biliary access point can be influenced by the degree of intrahepatic ductal dilation

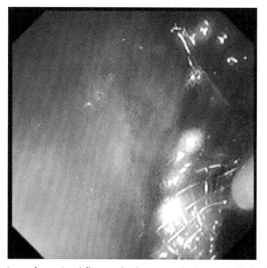

Fig. 5. Endoscopic view of proximal flange deployment during a choledochoduodenostomy.

on cross-sectional imaging (confirmed by EUS). If there is intrahepatic dilation, HGS is performed as the procedure of choice; if inadequate dilation or an HGS is unsuccessful, than a CDS should be pursued.[35] The authors demonstrated a technical success of 96% with a 10% AE rate.

Choice of stent in endoscopic ultrasound-guided biliary drainage

Several types of stents have been utilized for EUS-BD including plastic stents, covered or partially covered self-expanding metal stents (FCSEMS, PCSEMS, respectively), and LAMS(all of which are fully covered). FCSEMS and PCSEMS have largely replaced plastic stents in HGS due to the larger diameter and mechanism of deployment, yet stent migration remains a concern owing to the tubular shape, rigid properties, and larger size.[10] Partially covered stents with special hybrid design have been shown to reduce stent migration when HGS is performed.[27] A single-center prospective study enrolled 22 patients for EUS-HGS after failed ERCP using a newly dedicated PCSEMS with an anti-migratory system.[36] Technical success was achieved in all patients with no instances of stent migration. Anchoring with double pigtail plastic stents also helps decrease migration rates. There were no instances of stent migration in a large-scale single-center study of 205 HGS procedures where an FCSEMS with an anchoring plastic stent was used in the majority of cases.[33] The authors in this study noted that 21 patients required re-intervention for jaundice (17 of these individuals had hilar disease).[33] These interventions included percutaneous biliary drainage (n = 5), repeat endoscopic intervention that then required percutaneous biliary drainage (n = 5), endoscopic stent exchange/replacement, (n = 10) and one patient underwent a second HGS procedure to an undrained right intrahepatic system.[33]

LAMS have largely become the stent of choice for CDS, especially with the emergence of smaller diameter stents of 6 mm and 8 mm, due to the allowance for single-step fistula creation and stent deployment and biflanged shape to decrease migration rates. Initial studies noted a high rate of LAMS dysfunction occurring in 55% of cases, in which 9 patients required reintervention.[37] However, a more recent meta-analysis with 1081 patients undergoing EUS-CDS with LAMS found that the stent misdeployment rate was 5.8%.[37] LAMS are not used in HGS due to the longer length needed to bridge the left hepatic duct and stomach.

ENDOSCOPIC ULTRASOUND-GUIDED BILIARY DRAINAGE VERSUS PERCUTANEOUS TRANSHEPATIC BILIARY DRAINAGE

Comparative data favor EUS-BD as a less invasive option with fewer AEs and re-intervention rates compared with PTBD. A meta-analysis of 483 patients (9 studies) found that there was no difference in technical success, but EUS-BD was associated with better clinical success, lower rates of AEs, and fewer re-interventions when compared to PTBD.[38] An open label randomized control trial in South Korea compared EUS-BD (n = 34) to PTBD (n = 32), and showed that procedure-related AEs (8.8% vs 31.2%, P = .022) and unscheduled re-intervention rates (0.34 v 0.93, P=.03) were lower in the EUS-BD cohort.[39] Six other prospective and retrospective international comparative studies have shown similar findings.[40-45] Based on these studies, it is recommended to proceed with EUS-BD after failed ERCP when expertise is available.

ENDOSCOPIC ULTRASOUND-GUIDED BILIARY DRAINAGE VERSUS ENDOSCOPIC RETROGRADE CHOLANGIOPANCREATOGRAPHY

Several randomized controlled studies have compared EUS-BD as first-line therapy compared to conventional ERCP (**Table 1**).[46-50] One international randomized controlled

Table 1
Randomized controlled studies comparing outcomes of endoscopic ultrasound-guided biliary drainage and endoscopic retrograde cholangiopancreatography as first-line drainage

Author (Year)	Number of Patients (EUS-BD vs ERCP)	Technical Success (EUS-BD vs ERCP)	Clinical Success (EUS-BD vs ERCP)	Adverse Events	Stent Patency	Reintervention
Teoh et al,[48] 2023	155 (79 vs 76)	96.2% vs 76.3%	93.7% vs 90.8%	16.5% vs 17.1%	91.1% vs 88.1%	11.3% vs 12.7%
Chen et al,[46] 2023	144 (73 vs 71)	90.4% vs 83.1%	84.9% vs 85.9%	15.1% vs 16.9%	% not reported[b]	9.6% vs 9.9%
Paik et al,[50] 2018	125 (64 vs 61)	93.8% vs 90.2%	90.4% vs 94.5%	6.3% vs 19.7%	85.1% vs 48.9%	15.6% vs 42.6%
Park et al,[47] 2018	28 (14 vs 14)	93% vs 100%	100% vs 93%	31%[a]	69%[a]	n/a
Bang et al,[49] 2018	67 (34 vs 33)	90.9% vs 94.1%	97% vs 91.2%	14.7% vs 6.1%	n/a	3 vs 2.9%

[a] Study did not differentiate EUS-BD versus ERCP.
[b] Study reported mean stent patency time as 163.9 and 200.1 d.

trial compared EUS-BD (n = 73) and ERCP (n = 71) for malignant distal biliary obstruction. EUS-BD was associated with higher technical success (90.4% vs 83.1%) without major differences in stent dysfunction (9.6% vs 9.9%), AEs, or surgical outomes.[46] Another large multicenter, randomized controlled study of 155 patients (EUS-CDS 79, ERCP 76) found no difference in 1 year stent patency (91.1% vs 88.1%, P = .52).[48] EUS-CDS was associated with a higher technical success rate (96.2% vs 76.3%, P < .001) and shorter procedure time (10 vs 25 min, P < .001).[48] The authors suggested that EUS-CDS should be preferred when a difficult ERCP is anticipated, especially in cases of duodenal obstruction, distortion of the ampulla from malignant infiltration, and friability edematous mucosa in the second portion of the duodenum.[48] Additionally, EUS-BD may be preferable in patients at high risk for post-ERCP pancreatitis due to access of the biliary tree far from the pancreatic orifice. In a comparative study, EUS-BD demonstrated lower rates of AEs (6.3% vs 19.7%, P=.03), reintervention (15.6% vs 42.6%), and high rates of stent patency (85.1% vs 48.9%).[50] A large meta-analysis involving 7877 patients (155 studies) undergoing EUS-BD found that the overall AE rate, incidence of stent occlusion, and need for reintervention was 13.7%, 11%, and 16.2%, respectively.[51] It remains to be seen if EUS-BD will continue to expand into a first-line therapy for biliary obstruction over ERCP as additional data emerge.

PROCEDURAL LEARNING CURVE

EUS-BD is a specialized technique that is often limited to high-volume tertiary centers. The learning curve associated with this procedure has been studied, and there is a clear linear progression with procedure volume.[15,28,52–56] Two studies found that technical proficiency and mastery were achieved after 33 and 100 cases, respectively.[52,54] A large single-center study with one endoscopist performing 215 procedures over a 6.6 year period demonstrated a significant decrease in procedure-related AEs over time.[57] Another group found that a single endoscopist performing 101 procedures encountered 5 procedure-related deaths during the first 50 patients and only 1 among the last 51 patients.[28] Additionally, the volume of institution-based EUS screenings (≥436), fine needle aspirations (≥93), and drainage procedures (≥13) influenced EUS-BD outcomes.[55] A large systematic review with 42 studies found that studies published after 2013 reported higher success and lower AE rates and as such concluded that procedure volume is correlated with technical success.[58] Over time, increasing operator experience, dedicated procedural devices, and formalized training will likely result in more widespread adoption.

SURGERY AFTER ENDOSCOPIC ULTRASOUND-GUIDED BILIARY DRAINAGE

A proportion of patients with malignant biliary obstruction are candidates for surgical resection after biliary decompression. A common question is whether patients can proceed to surgery after undergoing EUS-BD as compared to conventional ERCP. Data on this subject are limited; however, recent studies suggest feasibility. One study compared patients who underwent curative surgery after having undergone EUS-BD to published data on outcomes of patients who underwent surgery after conventional ERCP and found that the overall (25% vs 55%) and major (15% vs 19%) surgical complications were lower in the EUS-BD group.[59] A more recent study of 145 patients who underwent hepatobiliary surgery after having undergone EUS-BD (n = 58) or ERCP (n = 87) found that EUS-BD was associated with fewer repeat endoscopic interventions, shorter duration between endoscopy and surgical intervention, higher rates of surgical clinical success, and shorter length of hospital stay after surgery.[60] The authors concluded that EUS-BD may actually be superior to conventional ERCP when performed prior to surgery, but should at minimum not impede patients from undergoing surgical intervention. However, additional data are needed.

ENDOSCOPIC ULTRASOUND BILIARY DRAINAGE IN BENIGN BILIARY DISEASE

EUS-BD can also be utilized in cases of benign biliary obstruction. Often, technique modifications with a 2-step EUS-guided approach have been used.[10] This typically first involves creation of an EUS-HGS that creates a portal to allow definitive antegrade stone extraction or biliary therapy such as antegrade stricture dilation.[61,62] If a metal stent is used, a long-term study (median follow-up of 749 days) found that scheduled plastic stent exchanges within 6 months was useful.[63]

While data are limited, a growing number of centers reported their experiences with promising results.[33,64,65] A recent meta-analysis of 14 studies with 329 patients reported a technical success, clinical success, and AE rate of 88%, 89%, and 19%, respectively.[66] Of note, AEs appear to be higher with EUS-BD compared to enteroscopy-assisted ERCP (6.5%).[67] One multicenter study compared repeat ERCP (n = 56) to EUS-BD (n = 36) in individuals who initially failed ERCP with normal foregut anatomy.[65] Technical success was 77.8% for EUS-BD and 86% in the repeat ERCP comparator group. The EUS-BD cohort experienced significantly higher rates of AEs (27.8% vs 8%), which emphasizes the importance for this procedure to be performed in high-volume centers with extensive operator experience. The lack of dilated target bile ducts can make needle puncture and guidewire manipulation difficult. One single-center study of 85 patientsreported technical success in 78 patients.[33] The average intrahepatic duct diameter was 5.7 mm in the technically successful cases and 3.0 mm in failed cases. Moving forward, dedicated devices and standardized patient algorithms are needed to improve technical success and determine optimal patient selection factors.

SUMMARY

Since its introduction in 2001, EUS-BD techniques have shown to be effective for relief of biliary obstruction with high technical and clinical success rates. While EUS-BD was initially reserved as a rescue for cases of unsuccessful biliary cannulation or an inaccessible papilla due to anatomic constraints, it is now considered a preferred first-line approach for select cases, even for native biliary anatomy, when performed by experienced operators. As EUS-BD continues to gain widespread adoption, it will likely replace conventional salvage therapy with percutaneous drainage approaches owing to fewer adverse events and reinterventions, and may even become first-line therapy for malignant biliary obstruction over conventional ERCP.

CLINICS CARE POINTS

- EUS-BD has become an acceptable alternative therapy for biliary decompression when conventional ERCP is unsuccessful with improved outcomes compared to PTBD.
- In malignant biliary obstruction, EUS-BD is proven non-inferior and possibly superior to conventional ERCP.
- EUS-BD can be performed via an intrahepatic or extrahepatic approach, and stenting can be performed via a rendezvous approach, antegrade placement, or transluminal placement via hepaticogastrostomy or choledochoduodenostomy. No consensus exists on which technique is superior and approach should be individualized.
- Procedural complexity and lack of dedicated procedural equipment have been limiting factors to the widespread application of these techniques.

- EUS-BD prior to surgical resection seems efficacious and safe; further confirmatory studies are needed.

DISCLOSURES

Dr A. Canakis has no disclosures. Dr A. Tyberg has done consulting work for Boston Scientific, Medtronic, Ambu Inc, and Microtech.

REFERENCES

1. Cennamo V, Fuccio L, Zagari RM, et al. Can early precut implementation reduce endoscopic retrograde cholangiopancreatography-related complication risk? Meta-analysis of randomized controlled trials. Endoscopy 2010;42(5):381–8.
2. Halttunen J, Meisner S, Aabakken L, et al. Difficult cannulation as defined by a prospective study of the Scandinavian Association for Digestive Endoscopy (SADE) in 907 ERCPs. Scand J Gastroenterol 2014;49(6):752–8.
3. Dumonceau JM, Tringali A, Papanikolaou IS, et al. Endoscopic biliary stenting: indications, choice of stents, and results: European Society of Gastrointestinal Endoscopy (ESGE) Clinical Guideline - Updated October 2017. Endoscopy 2018;50(9):910–30.
4. Testoni PA, Mariani A, Aabakken L, et al. Papillary cannulation and sphincterotomy techniques at ERCP: European Society of Gastrointestinal Endoscopy (ESGE) Clinical Guideline. Endoscopy 2016;48(7):657–83.
5. Canakis A, Kahaleh M. Endoscopic palliation of malignant biliary obstruction. World J Gastrointest Endosc 2022;14(10):581–96.
6. Inamdar S, Slattery E, Bhalla R, et al. Comparison of Adverse Events for Endoscopic vs Percutaneous Biliary Drainage in the Treatment of Malignant Biliary Tract Obstruction in an Inpatient National Cohort. JAMA Oncol 2016;2(1):112–7.
7. Wang L, Lin N, Xin F, et al. A systematic review of the comparison of the incidence of seeding metastasis between endoscopic biliary drainage and percutaneous transhepatic biliary drainage for resectable malignant biliary obstruction. World J Surg Oncol 2019;17:116.
8. Mukai S, Itoi T, Baron TH, et al. Indications and techniques of biliary drainage for acute cholangitis in updated Tokyo Guidelines 2018. J Hepato-Biliary-Pancreatic Sci 2017;24(10):537–49.
9. Giovannini M, Moutardier V, Pesenti C, et al. Endoscopic ultrasound-guided bilioduodenal anastomosis: a new technique for biliary drainage. Endoscopy 2001; 33(10):898–900.
10. Canakis A, Baron TH. Relief of biliary obstruction: choosing between endoscopic ultrasound and endoscopic retrograde cholangiopancreatography. BMJ Open Gastroenterol 2020;7(1):e000428.
11. Mallery S, Matlock J, Freeman ML. EUS-guided rendezvous drainage of obstructed biliary and pancreatic ducts: Report of 6 cases. Gastrointest Endosc 2004;59(1):100–7.
12. Kahaleh M, Hernandez AJ, Tokar J, et al. Interventional EUS-guided cholangiography: evaluation of a technique in evolution. Gastrointest Endosc 2006; 64(1):52–9.
13. Yoon SB, Yang MJ, Shin DW, et al. Endoscopic ultrasound-rendezvous versus percutaneous-endoscopic rendezvous endoscopic retrograde cholangiopancreatography for bile duct access: Systematic review and meta-analysis. Dig

Endosc Off J Jpn Gastroenterol Endosc Soc 2023. https://doi.org/10.1111/den. 14636. Published online July 11.

14. Tsuchiya T, Itoi T, Sofuni A, et al. Endoscopic ultrasonography-guided rendezvous technique. Dig Endosc 2016;28(S1):96–101.

15. Hara K, Yamao K, Mizuno N, et al. Endoscopic ultrasonography-guided biliary drainage: Who, when, which, and how? World J Gastroenterol 2016;22(3): 1297–303.

16. van Wanrooij RLJ, Bronswijk M, Kunda R, et al. Therapeutic endoscopic ultrasound: European Society of Gastrointestinal Endoscopy (ESGE) Technical Review. Endoscopy 2022;54(3):310–32.

17. Artifon ELA, Safatle-Ribeiro AV, Ferreira FC, et al. EUS-guided antegrade transhepatic placement of a self-expandable metal stent in hepatico-jejunal anastomosis. JOP J Pancreas 2011;12(6):610–3.

18. Iwashita T, Yasuda I, Doi S, et al. Endoscopic ultrasound-guided antegrade treatments for biliary disorders in patients with surgically altered anatomy. Dig Dis Sci 2013;58(8):2417–22.

19. Nguyen-Tang T, Binmoeller KF, Sanchez-Yague A, et al. Endoscopic ultrasound (EUS)-guided transhepatic anterograde self-expandable metal stent (SEMS) placement across malignant biliary obstruction. Endoscopy 2010;42(3):232–6.

20. Shah SL, Perez-Miranda M, Kahaleh M, et al. Updates in Therapeutic Endoscopic Ultrasonography. J Clin Gastroenterol 2018;52(9):765–72.

21. Park DH, Jang JW, Lee SS, et al. EUS-guided transhepatic antegrade balloon dilation for benign bilioenteric anastomotic strictures in a patient with hepaticojejunostomy. Gastrointest Endosc 2012;75(3):692–3.

22. Park DH, Jeong SU, Lee BU, et al. Prospective evaluation of a treatment algorithm with enhanced guidewire manipulation protocol for EUS-guided biliary drainage after failed ERCP (with video). Gastrointest Endosc 2013;78(1):91–101.

23. Ogura T, Chiba Y, Masuda D, et al. Comparison of the clinical impact of endoscopic ultrasound-guided choledochoduodenostomy and hepaticogastrostomy for bile duct obstruction with duodenal obstruction. Endoscopy 2016;48(2): 156–63.

24. Tyberg A, Napoleon B, Robles-Medranda C, et al. Hepaticogastrostomy versus choledochoduodenostomy: An international multicenter study on their long-term patency. Endosc Ultrasound 2022;11(1):38–43.

25. Artifon ELA, Marson FP, Gaidhane M, et al. Hepaticogastrostomy or choledochoduodenostomy for distal malignant biliary obstruction after failed ERCP: is there any difference? Gastrointest Endosc 2015;81(4):950–9.

26. Khashab MA, Messallam AA, Penas I, et al. International multicenter comparative trial of transluminal EUS-guided biliary drainage via hepatogastrostomy vs. choledochoduodenostomy approaches. Endosc Int Open 2016;4(2):E175–81.

27. Cho DH, Lee SS, Oh D, et al. Long-term outcomes of a newly developed hybrid metal stent for EUS-guided biliary drainage (with videos). Gastrointest Endosc 2017;85(5):1067–75.

28. Poincloux L, Rouquette O, Buc E, et al. Endoscopic ultrasound-guided biliary drainage after failed ERCP: cumulative experience of 101 procedures at a single center. Endoscopy 2015;47(9):794–801.

29. Kawakubo K, Isayama H, Kato H, et al. Multicenter retrospective study of endoscopic ultrasound-guided biliary drainage for malignant biliary obstruction in Japan. J Hepato-Biliary-Pancreatic Sci 2014;21(5):328–34.

30. Minaga K, Ogura T, Shiomi H, et al. Comparison of the efficacy and safety of endoscopic ultrasound-guided choledochoduodenostomy and hepaticogastrostomy

for malignant distal biliary obstruction: Multicenter, randomized, clinical trial. Dig Endosc Off J Jpn Gastroenterol Endosc Soc 2019;31(5):575–82.

31. Yamazaki H, Yamashita Y, Shimokawa T, et al. Endoscopic ultrasound-guided hepaticogastrostomy versus choledochoduodenostomy for malignant biliary obstruction: A meta-analysis. DEN Open. 2024;4(1):e274.

32. Guo J, Giovannini M, Sahai AV, et al. A multi-institution consensus on how to perform EUS-guided biliary drainage for malignant biliary obstruction. Endosc Ultrasound 2018;7(6):356–65.

33. Hathorn KE, Canakis A, Baron TH. EUS-guided transhepatic biliary drainage: a large single-center U.S. experience. Gastrointest Endosc 2022;95(3):443–51.

34. Vila JJ, Pérez-Miranda M, Vazquez-Sequeiros E, et al. Initial experience with EUS-guided cholangiopancreatography for biliary and pancreatic duct drainage: a Spanish national survey. Gastrointest Endosc 2012;76(6):1133–41.

35. Tyberg A, Desai AP, Kumta NA, et al. EUS-guided biliary drainage after failed ERCP: a novel algorithm individualized based on patient anatomy. Gastrointest Endosc 2016;84(6):941–6.

36. Anderloni A, Fugazza A, Spadaccini M, et al. Feasibility and safety of a new dedicated biliary stent for EUS-guided hepaticogastrostomy: The FIT study (with video). Endosc Ultrasound 2023;12(1):59–63.

37. Armellini E, Metelli F, Anderloni A, et al. Lumen-apposing-metal stent misdeployment in endoscopic ultrasound-guided drainages: A systematic review focusing on issues and rescue management. World J Gastroenterol 2023;29(21):3341–61.

38. Sharaiha RZ, Khan MA, Kamal F, et al. Efficacy and safety of EUS-guided biliary drainage in comparison with percutaneous biliary drainage when ERCP fails: a systematic review and meta-analysis. Gastrointest Endosc 2017;85(5):904–14.

39. Lee TH, Choi JH, Park DH, et al. Similar Efficacies of Endoscopic Ultrasound-guided Transmural and Percutaneous Drainage for Malignant Distal Biliary Obstruction. Clin Gastroenterol Hepatol Off Clin Pract J Am Gastroenterol Assoc 2016;14(7):1011–9.e3.

40. Khashab MA, Valeshabad AK, Afghani E, et al. A comparative evaluation of EUS-guided biliary drainage and percutaneous drainage in patients with distal malignant biliary obstruction and failed ERCP. Dig Dis Sci 2015;60(2):557–65.

41. Schmitz D, Valiente CT, Dollhopf M, et al. Percutaneous transhepatic or endoscopic ultrasound-guided biliary drainage in malignant distal bile duct obstruction using a self-expanding metal stent: Study protocol for a prospective European multicenter trial (PUMa trial). PLoS One 2022;17(10):e0275029.

42. Sharaiha RZ, Kumta NA, Desai AP, et al. Endoscopic ultrasound-guided biliary drainage versus percutaneous transhepatic biliary drainage: predictors of successful outcome in patients who fail endoscopic retrograde cholangiopancreatography. Surg Endosc 2016;30(12):5500–5.

43. Artifon ELA, Aparicio D, Paione JB, et al. Biliary drainage in patients with unresectable, malignant obstruction where ERCP fails: endoscopic ultrasonography-guided choledochoduodenostomy versus percutaneous drainage. J Clin Gastroenterol 2012;46(9):768–74.

44. Bapaye A, Dubale N, Aher A. Comparison of endosonography-guided vs. percutaneous biliary stenting when papilla is inaccessible for ERCP. United Eur Gastroenterol J 2013;1(4):285–93.

45. Marx M, Caillol F, Autret A, et al. EUS-guided hepaticogastrostomy in patients with obstructive jaundice after failed or impossible endoscopic retrograde drainage: A multicenter, randomized phase II Study. Endosc Ultrasound 2022;11(6):495–502.

46. Chen YI, Sahai A, Donatelli G, et al. Endoscopic Ultrasound-Guided Biliary Drainage of First Intent With a Lumen-Apposing Metal Stent vs Endoscopic Retrograde Cholangiopancreatography in Malignant Distal Biliary Obstruction: A Multicenter Randomized Controlled Study (ELEMENT Trial). Gastroenterology 2023. S0016-5085(23)04877-1.

47. Park JK, Woo YS, Noh DH, et al. Efficacy of EUS-guided and ERCP-guided biliary drainage for malignant biliary obstruction: prospective randomized controlled study. Gastrointest Endosc 2018;88(2):277–82.

48. Teoh AYB, Napoleon B, Kunda R, et al. EUS-Guided Choledocho-duodenostomy Using Lumen Apposing Stent Versus ERCP With Covered Metallic Stents in Patients With Unresectable Malignant Distal Biliary Obstruction: A Multicenter Randomized Controlled Trial (DRA-MBO Trial). Gastroenterology 2023;165(2): 473–82.e2.

49. Bang JY, Navaneethan U, Hasan M, et al. Stent placement by EUS or ERCP for primary biliary decompression in pancreatic cancer: a randomized trial (with videos). Gastrointest Endosc 2018;88(1):9–17.

50. Paik WH, Lee TH, Park DH, et al. EUS-Guided Biliary Drainage Versus ERCP for the Primary Palliation of Malignant Biliary Obstruction: A Multicenter Randomized Clinical Trial. Am J Gastroenterol 2018;113(7):987–97.

51. Giri S, Mohan BP, Jearth V, et al. Adverse Events with Endoscopic Ultrasound-guided Biliary Drainage: A Systematic Review and Meta-analysis. Gastrointest Endosc 2023. S0016-5107(23)02706-2.

52. Oh D, Park DH, Song TJ, et al. Optimal biliary access point and learning curve for endoscopic ultrasound-guided hepaticogastrostomy with transmural stenting. Ther Adv Gastroenterol 2017;10(1):42–53.

53. Tyberg A, Kats D, Choi A, et al. Endoscopic Ultrasound Guided Gastroenterostomy: What Is the Learning Curve? J Clin Gastroenterol 2021;55(8):691–3.

54. Tyberg A, Mishra A, Cheung M, et al. Learning curve for EUS-guided biliary drainage: What have we learned? Endosc Ultrasound 2020;9(6):392–6.

55. Sagami R, Mizukami K, Okamoto K, et al. Experience-Related Factors in the Success of Beginner Endoscopic Ultrasound-Guided Biliary Drainage: A Multicenter Study. J Clin Med 2023;12(6):2393.

56. Attasaranya S, Netinasunton N, Jongboonyanuparp T, et al. The Spectrum of Endoscopic Ultrasound Intervention in Biliary Diseases: A Single Center's Experience in 31 Cases. Gastroenterol Res Pract 2012;2012:680753.

57. Hathorn KE, Bazarbashi AN, Sack JS, et al. EUS-guided biliary drainage is equivalent to ERCP for primary treatment of malignant distal biliary obstruction: a systematic review and meta-analysis. Endosc Int Open 2019;7(11): E1432–41.

58. Wang K, Zhu J, Xing L, et al. Assessment of efficacy and safety of EUS-guided biliary drainage: a systematic review. Gastrointest Endosc 2016;83(6):1218–27.

59. Tyberg A, Ventre S, Abdelqader A, et al. 3526980 Curative surgery after EUS-guided biliary drainage: an international multicenter feasibilty study. Gastrointest Endosc 2021;93(6):AB266.

60. Tyberg A, Sarkar A, Shahid HM, et al. EUS-Guided Biliary Drainage Versus ERCP in Malignant Biliary Obstruction Before Hepatobiliary Surgery: An International Multicenter Comparative Study. J Clin Gastroenterol 2023;57(9):962–6.

61. James TW, Fan YC, Baron TH. EUS-guided hepaticoenterostomy as a portal to allow definitive antegrade treatment of benign biliary diseases in patients with surgically altered anatomy. Gastrointest Endosc 2018;88(3):547–54.

62. Miranda-García P, Gonzalez JM, Tellechea JI, et al. EUS hepaticogastrostomy for bilioenteric anastomotic strictures: a permanent access for repeated ambulatory dilations? Results from a pilot study. Endosc Int Open 2016; 4(4):E461–5.

63. Ogura T, Takenaka M, Shiomi H, et al. Long-term outcomes of EUS-guided transluminal stent deployment for benign biliary disease: Multicenter clinical experience (with videos). Endosc Ultrasound 2019;8(6):398–403.

64. Matsunami Y, Itoi T, Sofuni A, et al. EUS-guided hepaticoenterostomy with using a dedicated plastic stent for the benign pancreaticobiliary diseases: A single-center study of a large case series. Endosc Ultrasound 2021;10(4):294–304.

65. Bill JG, Ryou M, Hathorn KE, et al. Endoscopic ultrasound-guided biliary drainage in benign biliary pathology with normal foregut anatomy: a multicenter study. Surg Endosc 2022;36(2):1362–8.

66. Kamal F, Khan MA, Lee-Smith W, et al. Efficacy and safety of EUS-guided biliary drainage for benign biliary obstruction - A systematic review and meta-analysis. Endosc Ultrasound 2023;12(2):228–36.

67. Inamdar S, Slattery E, Sejpal DV, et al. Systematic review and meta-analysis of single-balloon enteroscopy-assisted ERCP in patients with surgically altered GI anatomy. Gastrointest Endosc 2015;82(1):9–19.

Endoscopic Ultrasound-Guided Pancreatic Duct Drainage

Judy A. Trieu, MD, MPH[a], Gulseren Seven, MD[b],
Todd H. Baron, MD[c],*

KEYWORDS

- Endoscopic ultrasound • EUS-guided pancreaticogastrostomy
- EUS-guided pancreatic rendezvous
- Endoscopic retrograde cholangiopancreatography • Pancreatic duct drainage

KEY POINTS

- Endoscopic ultrasound-guided pancreatic duct drainage (EUS-PDD) is a minimally invasive alternative to surgery for selected cases of pancreatic disease when conventional endoscopic retrograde pancreatography (ERP) fails or is not technically feasible, particularly in cases involving surgically altered foregut anatomy.
- Clinical success of EUS-PDD is comparable to that of surgical procedures and is associated with lower risks of adverse events; therefore, it should be considered before surgery.
- Because of the complexity of the technique and the risks of adverse events, EUS-PDD should be performed by endoscopists experienced in both therapeutic EUS-PDD and endoscopic retrograde cholangiopancreatography (ERCP) at tertiary referral centers specializing in pancreatic diseases.
- EUS-PDD should be performed with the support of well-trained surgeons and interventional radiologists in events of technical failure or severe adverse events.
- EUS-assisted pancreatic rendezvous (EUS-PRV) should be preferred in easily accessible papilla or anastomosis; otherwise, transmural EUS-guided pancreaticogastrostomy (EUS-PG) could be attempted first.

[a] Division of Gastroenterology, Washington University in St. Louis, 660 South Euclid Avenue, MSC 8124-21-427, St Louis, MO 63110, USA; [b] Division of Gastroenterology, Bezmialem Foundation University, Bezmialem Vakif University School of Medicine, Adnan Menderes Boulevard, Fatih, Istanbul 34093, Turkey; [c] Division of Gastroenterology and Hepatology, University of North Carolina, 130 Mason Farm Road, Bioinformatics Building CB# 7080, Chapel Hill, NC 27599-7080, USA
* Corresponding author. 130 Mason Farm Road, CB 7080, Chapel Hill, NC 27599.
E-mail address: todd_baron@med.unc.edu
Twitter: @TrieuMD (J.A.T.); @EndoTx (T.H.B.)

Gastrointest Endoscopy Clin N Am 34 (2024) 501–510
https://doi.org/10.1016/j.giec.2024.02.002
1052-5157/24/© 2024 Elsevier Inc. All rights reserved.

giendo.theclinics.com

INTRODUCTION

Endoscopic retrograde pancreatography (ERP) has been the primary technique for endoscopic decompression of the pancreatic duct (PD). Retrograde papillary access by experts is successful in 90% to 97% of procedures performed for patients with native anatomy.[1] However, PD access can be difficult or not feasible because of tight strictures or stones, tortuous duct variants that may hinder deep cannulation, surgically altered foregut anatomy, luminal obstruction or in situ duodenal stents preventing access to the major papilla or minor papilla, or disconnection of the PD. The technical success of conventional ERP for PD access can be as low as 8% after the Whipple procedure.[2] Surgical decompression of the pancreatic duct in chronic pancreatitis is effective, with high technical and clinical success rates.[3] However, endoscopic ultrasound-guided PD drainage (EUS-PDD) has emerged as an approach to obviate surgery and provide definitive therapy for nonsurgical candidates. EUS-PDD is achieved by accessing the PD with a wire to either facilitate transpapillary ERP therapy in EUS-assisted pancreatic rendezvous (EUS-PRV)[4–7] or transmural PD drainage with EUS-guided pancreaticogastrostomy (EUS-PG).[8–10] Because the majority of transmural EUS-guided PD drainage occurs from the stomach, the term "EUS-PG" is used in this review; however, rarely, EUS-pancreaticoenterostomies are performed.

In 1995, Harada and colleagues first reported EUS-guided pancreatography in a patient with a pylorus-preserving pancreaticoduodenectomy after ERCP and percutaneous pancreatography failed to reach the pancreatic anastomosis and poor visualization by transabdominal ultrasound, respectively.[11] In 2002, Francis and colleagues described the technique and feasibility of EUS-PG to decompress the PD in 4 patients with chronic pancreatitis after failed ERCP.[12] Bataille and colleagues reported the first EUS-PRV for a patient with a suprapapillary PD stricture.[4] Currently, despite its advances, EUS-PDD remains a challenging and infrequently performed technique to gain access to the PD when ERCP fails or is not feasible because of altered anatomy, even at specialized centers for advanced endoscopic procedures. Although EUS-PDD has been shown to be effective, it has not been widely adopted because of the high rates of adverse events even among experienced endoscopists. This review describes the role and current status of EUS-PDD in clinical practice.

INDICATIONS FOR ENDOSCOPIC ULTRASOUND-GUIDED PANCREATIC DUCT DRAINAGE

The current guidelines recommend ERP as the first choice of endoscopic therapy for PD decompression.[13,14] EUS-PDD should be considered a salvage procedure after the technical failure of retrograde pancreatic access or as an alternative to enteroscopy-assisted ERCP (E-ERCP), for patients with inaccessible papilla such as in altered anatomy. If ERP fails, then EUS-PRV should be considered if the papilla or anastomosis is easily accessible. EUS-PG should be preferred for patients with altered anatomy or for cases for which the guidewire cannot pass an obstruction.

The aims of these procedures are to decompress the pancreatic ductal pressure that can cause pain and/or pancreatitis and to restore drainage of the pancreatic fluid to the gastrointestinal lumen. Patients should have clear clinical indications for these procedures, such as disabling, typical pancreatic pain, or acute relapsing pancreatitis associated with obstruction (stones, strictures) from chronic pancreatitis or postsurgical pancreatic anastomosis. Rarely, EUS-PDD alone or in conjunction with conventional ERP can treat peri-pancreatic collections and fistulas due to disconnected or disrupted pancreatic ducts.[15]

CONTRAINDICATIONS

Patient-related contraindications include severe coagulopathy or hemodynamic instability that may preclude adequate sedation.[16] Other relative contraindications include nondilated PD (unable to visualize clearly) by EUS and intervening vasculature.[1] Intravenous secretin given intraprocedurally may be considered to increase the PD size. Multiple-focal PD strictures are considered contraindications;[17] however, if the strictures can be clearly identified on prior imaging (eg, magnetic resonance cholangiopancreatography), then EUS-PDD with transmural puncture upstream from the culprit strictures may be feasible.

TECHNICAL ASPECTS

In addition to the standard recommendations for endoscopic procedures provided by the guidelines, EUS-PDD should be performed under general anesthesia and using CO_2 insufflation while the patient is in the supine or prone position. Rectal nonsteroidal antiinflammatory prophylaxis is recommended, although data are lacking.[13] There are no data supporting the use of antibiotics, but they may be beneficial in events of ductal leakage resulting in peritonitis.[13,17]

Pancreatic Duct Access

A linear echoendoscope is positioned in the stomach or duodenal bulb to visualize the upstream, dilated PD (**Fig. 1A, B**), which can be confirmed with fluoroscopic positioning of the echoendoscope (**Fig. 2**). Intravenous secretin can be used to enhance PD diameter and facilitate needle access into the PD. A 19-gauge needle is typically used, which allows the passage of guidewires up to 0.035″ diameter. While a 0.035″ wire is often preferred because of its stiffness and stability, an available 0.025″ wire with equal stiffness (VisiGlide, Olympus Corporation, Center Valley, PA) is our first choice. For instances of repeated failure to achieve PD access with a fibrotic pancreas, a 22-gauge needle, which allows the passage of 0.021-inch and 0.018-inch guidewires, can be used for further attempts. After confirming access to the PD (**Fig. 3A, B**), the needle is flushed with saline to prevent difficulty with guidewire advancement. A 450 cm long guidewire is inserted into the needle and advanced into the PD toward the papilla or anastomosis (**Fig. 4A, B**). Manipulation of the guidewire can be difficult because any "pull-back" movement can induce shearing of the wire, which occurs more often with a smaller caliber needle. Shearing of the guidewire can result in fragmentation, leading to pancreatitis, PD leaks, bleeding, and perforation.[17]

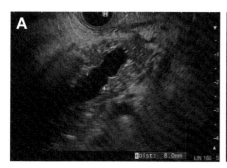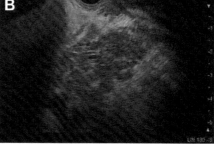

Fig. 1. EUS image of a dilated pancreatic duct from a downstream stricture of a dilated (A) and a minimally dilated pancreatic duct (B) in chronic pancreatitis.

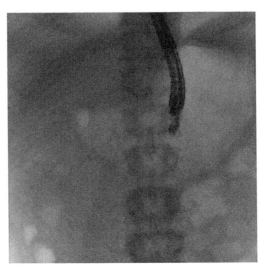

Fig. 2. Fluoroscopic demonstration of echoendoscope position to ensure the needle trajectory is toward the papilla or anastomosis.

Endoscopic Ultrasound-Guided Pancreatic Rendezvous

In EUS-PRV, the wire is advanced across the papilla or surgical anastomosis. Hydrophilic wires have a better ability to traverse the PD, particularly across strictures and stones. Then, the echoendoscope is exchanged for a duodenoscope or pediatric colonoscope, while the guidewire remains in place for subsequent ERP. A snare or grasper is used to grip the guidewire emerging from the papilla or anastomosis and the guidewire is pulled through the scope. Cannulation of the PD over or next to the guidewire is performed. After cannulation, additional therapy such as dilation, extraction of stones/debris, and placement of stents are performed accordingly. As with all rendezvous procedures, there is a risk of losing guidewire access, and of crossing guidewire.

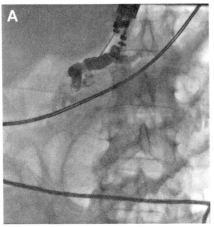
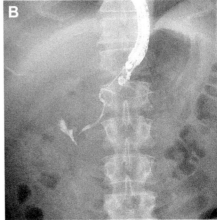

Fig. 3. Pancreatography to delineate the pancreatic duct anatomy in pancreatic duct obstruction (*A, B*).

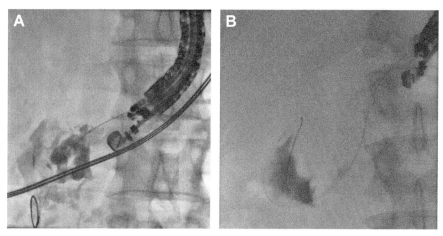

Fig. 4. Wire was advanced beyond the papilla using a hydrophilic 0.025 cm by 450 cm wire (*A, B*).

Endoscopic Ultrasound-Guided Pancreaticogastrostomy

In EUS-PG, transmural drainage can also be achieved from the duodenal bulb in select cases, but the endoscopic anastomosis is primarily performed from the stomach. Once wire access is gained as described above, either mechanical or cautery-based devices are used over the guidewire to create a fistulous tract. These exchanges are associated with the risk of guidewire dislodgement. A tapered dilating catheter (we use a 5-4-3 tip catheter (Contour, BSCI, Marlborough, MA), which accepts a well-lubricated 0.025″ VisiGlide wire) to then allow passage of a 4-mm hydrostatic balloon are used for mechanical dilation (**Fig. 5**A, B). A needle knife or 6-Fr cystotome is used to apply pure cutting current when these mechanical dilation fails. Mechanical dilation is associated with a slightly higher technical success compared with cystotome,[18] but it can be difficult to advance the balloon through the tract and fibrotic pancreatic parenchyma while maintaining scope position in the stomach.

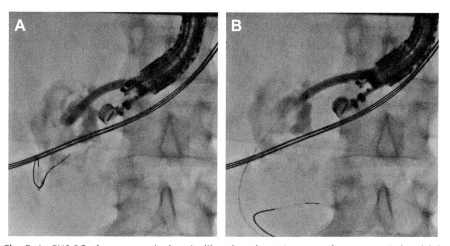

Fig. 5. In EUS-PG, the pancreatic duct is dilated at the stricture at the pancreatic head (*A*) and the transmural gastric puncture site (*B*).

A 6-Fr cystotome, only recently available in the United States, is easier to manipulate than other diathermic devices; however, the lack of stability of the endoscope in the stomach remains a major issue regardless of which device is used. Cautery-based devices can cause thermal injury to the surrounding tissues. Pure cutting current during passage through the wall and pancreatic parenchyma facilitates easier access and less current diffusion, whereas combined cutting-coagulation currents are less effective and have more uncontrolled current diffusion leading to a higher risk of injury to an adjacent vessel. Both dilation and cautery can result in a PD leak and free peritoneal air. Thereafter, one or more 7-Fr or 5-Fr plastic stents are placed transmurally. All PD stents should be positioned toward the head of the pancreas. If the guidewire passes transpapillary or transanastomosis to create a gastropancreaticoenterostomy (ring drainage), a double pigtail stent is preferred to reduce the risk of migration (**Fig. 6**A, B). After 1 month, the tract should be mature for further interventions, such as dilation, stent revision, or direct pancreatoscopy, as needed. Fully covered self-expandable metal stents can also be used and may decrease the risk of PD leak (see **Fig. 6**A, B); however, specific adverse events (ie, side branch occlusion, migration, ductal injuries) should be considered and no advantages over plastic stents have been shown.[19] Uncovered self-expandable metal stents are not indicated for EUS-PDD. In patients who are deemed to be stent-dependent (ie, untraversable or refractory downstream stricture), the single stent can be replaced after tract maturation with 2 side-by-side 7-Fr or 5-Fr stents (usually straight rather than single pigtail) indefinitely to ensure the longevity of the tract.

For patients with PD strictures or stones secondary to chronic pancreatitis, EUS-PRV allows physiologic drainage of pancreatic secretions through the papilla or surgical anastomosis to the lumen. However, EUS-PG is a viable option in failed rendezvous ERP or in technically challenging altered anatomy, such as post-Whipple procedure (**Fig. 7**A–D).

CLINICAL OUTCOMES

At expert centers performing EUS-PDD, technical success ranged from 79% to 100%.[7,8,19–21] In a systematic review, altered anatomy and method of tract dilation

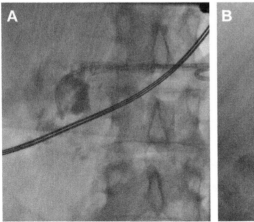
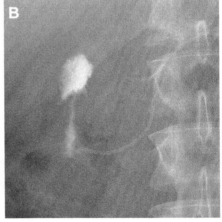

Fig. 6. A fully covered self-expandable metal stent with a coaxial plastic stent can be used for EUS-PG in moderately to severely dilated PD (*A*); otherwise, a plastic stent is typically used to maintain the EUS-PG tract (*B*).

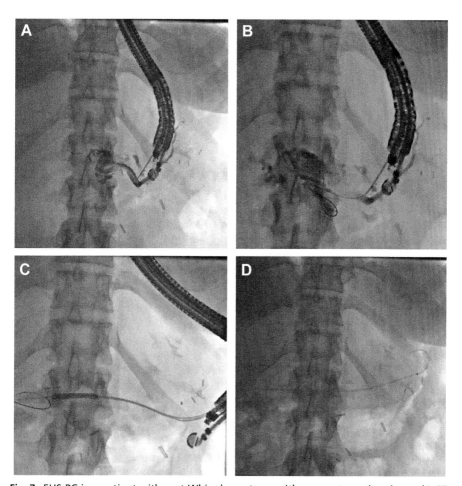

Fig. 7. EUS-PG in a patient with post-Whipple anatomy with an anastomotic stricture (*A*, PD access with pancreatogram; *B*, wire access with trajectory toward the anastomosis; *C*, mechanical dilation of the anastomotic stricture; *D*, plastic stent placed to maintain EUS-PG tract).

seemed to contribute to the variance in technical success.[18] The presence or recurrence of cancer was found to be associated with technical failure in one small cohort in post-Whipple and patients with chronic pancreatitis undergoing EUS-PDD.[8]

Reported clinical successes also ranged from 79% to 100%.[7,8,19–21] In a small cohort of EUS-PG only to treat PD strictures, mean PD size and abdominal pain score significantly decreased over a mean follow-up of 14 months.[22] EUS-PDD either as a means for further intervention (eg, stricture treatment, stone removal) or as definitive therapy yielded durable long-term clinical results. Greater than 69% of the cohorts followed for over a median of 1 year were pain-free.[8,21,23,24] Chandan, and colleagues remarked that patients with chronic pancreatitis may undergo other methods of pain management, such as celiac plexus blocks and oral analgesic; therefore, unless controlled for, it would be difficult to associate the clinical success rate to EUS-PDD alone.[25]

In a subgroup analysis of a systematic review, EUS-PG drainage had higher pooled technical success and contributed to the variance in clinical success[18]; however, this may be biased as the studies included many patients who underwent EUS-PRV after failed EUS-PG. In another systematic review, neither the indication of procedure (chronic pancreatitis) nor the EUS-PDD method (EUS-PRV, EUS-PG) were associated with any clinical outcomes.[25] Kraftt and colleagues proposed that attempting EUS-PG with ring drainage (gastropancreaticoenterostomy) should be the goal of the index procedure if feasible because it may achieve greater technical success (more available guidewire tension for dilation and transmural stent deployment) and clinical success with dual drainage.[26]

ADVERSE EVENTS

Adverse events from EUS-PDD ranged from 12% to 35% in cohort studies[7,19,20,27]; similarly, in systematic reviews, pooled AEs ranged from 18% to 21%.[16,18,25,28] The most common AE across the studies was abdominal pain followed by pancreatitis. Other reported adverse events included bleeding, perforation/pneumoperitoneum, pancreatic duct leak, and infection.[25] Long-term AEs were typically stent-related, leading to recurrent symptoms of pain and/or pancreatitis. Stent occlusion and/or migration occurred in up to 50% of patients,[8] requiring re-intervention in 15.2% in one systematic review of studies.[25] Studies had not shown any differences in AEs based on the EUS-PDD method (EUS-PRV vs EUS-PG).

The rates of AEs tend to be higher in EUS-PDD procedures compared with other EUS-guided interventions. In a large cohort study, the technical success rates increased from 41% in the first third of procedures to 76% in the final third of procedures. The learning curve for EUS-PDD was steep, with 80-min efficiency achieved at the 27th case and mastery at the 40th case.[29] However, it should be noted that these studies reflect high-volume centers; therefore, technical success, efficiency, and mastery may take longer to reach in other settings.

SUMMARY

EUS-PDD remains a challenging but feasible alternative when conventional ERP fails, with a technical failure rate up to 30%, even when performed by experienced endoscopists and an AE rate of approximately 20%. Long-term studies show durable pain relief for the majority of patients. Stent migration and occlusion rates are high; however, more longitudinal studies are required to better understand stent-related outcomes as well as factors contributing to stent malfunction.

Because of its technical complexity and relatively high AEs, EUS-PDD should be performed at advanced tertiary care centers by experienced operators. EUS-PRV should be attempted if the papilla or anastomosis is easily accessible; otherwise, EUS-PG is a comparable alternative. A multidisciplinary approach that considers the patient's anatomy, indication of EUS-PDD, long-term goals, and patient's preference should be performed to allow optimal management.

CLINICS CARE POINTS

- The 2 types of EUS-guided pancreatic duct drainage (EUS-PDD) are EUS-assisted pancreatic rendezvous (EUS-PRV) and EUS-guided pancreaticogastrostomy (EUS-PG).
- EUS-PDD is indicated to treat decompress the pancreatic duct after inability to access the papilla or surgical anastomosis.

- Contraindications for EUS-PDD include severe coagulopathy, hemodynamically unstable patients, nondilated PDs, and intervening vessels in the needle trajectory.
- Although technical and clinical successes are promising, rates of adverse events are relatively high among EUS-guided interventions, even among expert endoscopists.
- Because of the complexity of EUS-PDD, a multidisciplinary approach including surgery, interventional radiology, and the patient should be used.

DISCLOSURES

The article has been read and approved by all the authors. G. Seven and J.A. Trieu have nothing to disclose. T.H. Baron is a consultant and speaker for Ambu, Boston Scientific, Cook Endoscopy, Medtronic, Olympus America, ConMed, and W.L. Gore.

REFERENCES

1. Khan Z, Hayat U, Moraveji S, et al. EUS-guided pancreatic ductal intervention: A comprehensive literature review. Endosc Ultrasound 2021;10(2):98–102.
2. Chahal P, Baron TH, Topazian MD, et al. Endoscopic retrograde cholangiopancreatography in post-Whipple patients. Endoscopy 2006;38(12):1241–5.
3. Cahen DL, Gouma DJ, Nio Y, et al. Endoscopic versus surgical drainage of the pancreatic duct in chronic pancreatitis. N Engl J Med 2007;356(7):676–84.
4. Bataille L, Deprez P. A new application for therapeutic EUS: main pancreatic duct drainage with a "pancreatic rendezvous technique". Gastrointest Endosc 2002; 55(6):740–3.
5. Mallery S, Matlock J, Freeman ML. EUS-guided rendezvous drainage of obstructed biliary and pancreatic ducts: Report of 6 cases. Gastrointest Endosc 2004;59(1):100–7.
6. Will U, Meyer F, Manger T, et al. Endoscopic ultrasound-assisted rendezvous maneuver to achieve pancreatic duct drainage in obstructive chronic pancreatitis. Endoscopy 2005;37(2):171–3.
7. Motomura D, Irani S, Larsen M, et al. Multicenter retrospective cohort of EUS-guided anterograde pancreatic duct access. Endosc Int Open 2023;11(4): E358–65.
8. Ergun M, Aouattah T, Gillain C, et al. Endoscopic ultrasound-guided transluminal drainage of pancreatic duct obstruction: long-term outcome. Endoscopy 2011; 43(6):518–25.
9. Shah JN, Marson F, Weilert F, et al. Single-operator, single-session EUS-guided anterograde cholangiopancreatography in failed ERCP or inaccessible papilla. Gastrointest Endosc 2012;75(1):56–64.
10. Will U, Fueldner F, Thieme AK, et al. Transgastric pancreatography and EUS-guided drainage of the pancreatic duct. J Hepatobiliary Pancreat Surg 2007; 14(4):377–82.
11. Harada N, Kouzu T, Arima M, et al. Endoscopic ultrasound-guided pancreatography: a case report. Endoscopy 1995;27(8):612–5.
12. Francois E, Kahaleh M, Giovannini M, et al. EUS-guided pancreaticogastrostomy. Gastrointest Endosc 2002;56(1):128–33.
13. van Wanrooij RLJ, Bronswijk M, Kunda R, et al. Therapeutic endoscopic ultrasound: European Society of Gastrointestinal Endoscopy (ESGE) Technical Review. Endoscopy 2022;54(3):310–32.

14. van der Merwe SW, van Wanrooij RLJ, Bronswijk M, et al. Therapeutic endoscopic ultrasound: European Society of Gastrointestinal Endoscopy (ESGE) Guideline. Endoscopy 2022;54(2):185–205.
15. Ghandour B, Akshintala VS, Bejjani M, et al. A modified approach for endoscopic ultrasound-guided management of disconnected pancreatic duct syndrome via drainage of a communicating collection. Endoscopy 2022;54(9):917–9.
16. Fujii-Lau LL, Levy MJ. Endoscopic ultrasound-guided pancreatic duct drainage. J Hepatobiliary Pancreat Sci 2015;22(1):51–7.
17. Itoi T, Kasuya K, Sofuni A, et al. Endoscopic ultrasonography-guided pancreatic duct access: techniques and literature review of pancreatography, transmural drainage and rendezvous techniques. Dig Endosc 2013;25(3):241–52.
18. Bhurwal A, Tawadros A, Mutneja H, et al. EUS guided pancreatic duct decompression in surgically altered anatomy or failed ERCP - A systematic review, meta-analysis and meta-regression. Pancreatology 2021;21(5):990–1000.
19. Oh D., Park D.H., Cho M.K., et al., Feasibility and safety of a fully covered self-expandable metal stent with antimigration properties for EUS-guided pancreatic duct drainage: early and midterm outcomes (with video), Gastrointest Endosc, 83 (2), 2016, 366–373.e2.
20. Chen YI, Levy MJ, Moreels TG, et al. An international multicenter study comparing EUS-guided pancreatic duct drainage with enteroscopy-assisted endoscopic retrograde pancreatography after Whipple surgery. Gastrointest Endosc 2017;85(1):170–7.
21. Fujii LL, Topazian MD, Abu Dayyeh BK, et al. EUS-guided pancreatic duct intervention: outcomes of a single tertiary-care referral center experience. Gastrointest Endosc 2013;78(6):854–64.e1.
22. Kahaleh M, Hernandez AJ, Tokar J, et al. EUS-guided pancreaticogastrostomy: analysis of its efficacy to drain inaccessible pancreatic ducts. Gastrointest Endosc 2007;65(2):224–30.
23. Tessier G, Bories E, Arvanitakis M, et al. EUS-guided pancreatogastrostomy and pancreatobulbostomy for the treatment of pain in patients with pancreatic ductal dilatation inaccessible for transpapillary endoscopic therapy. Gastrointest Endosc 2007;65(2):233–41.
24. Kurihara T, Itoi T, Sofuni A, et al. Endoscopic ultrasonography-guided pancreatic duct drainage after failed endoscopic retrograde cholangiopancreatography in patients with malignant and benign pancreatic duct obstructions. Dig Endosc 2013;25(Suppl 2):109–16.
25. Chandan S, Mohan BP, Khan SR, et al. Efficacy and safety of endoscopic ultrasound-guided pancreatic duct drainage (EUS-PDD): A systematic review and meta-analysis of 714 patients. Endosc Int Open 2020;8(11):E1664–72.
26. Krafft MR, Croglio MP, James TW, et al. Endoscopic endgame for obstructive pancreatopathy: outcomes of anterograde EUS-guided pancreatic duct drainage. A dual-center study. Gastrointest Endosc 2020;92(5):1055–66.
27. Tyberg A, Sharaiha RZ, Kedia P, et al. EUS-guided pancreatic drainage for pancreatic strictures after failed ERCP: a multicenter international collaborative study. Gastrointest Endosc 2017;85(1):164–9.
28. Basiliya K, Veldhuijzen G, Gerges C, et al. Endoscopic retrograde pancreatography-guided versus endoscopic ultrasound-guided technique for pancreatic duct cannulation in patients with pancreaticojejunostomy stenosis: a systematic literature review. Endoscopy 2021;53(3):266–76.
29. Tyberg A, Bodiwala V, Kedia P, et al. EUS-guided pancreatic drainage: A steep learning curve. Endosc Ultrasound 2020;9(3):175–9.

Transenteric Endoscopic Retrograde Cholangiopancreatography in Non-roux-en-Y Surgically Altered Anatomy

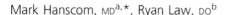

Mark Hanscom, MD[a],*, Ryan Law, DO[b]

KEYWORDS

- ERCP • Surgically altered anatomy • Endoscopic ultrasound • Whipple procedure
- Lumen-apposing metal stent • EUS-Guided transenteric ERCP (EDEE)

KEY POINTS

- ERCP is a challenging procedure in patients with surgically altered anatomy (SAA).
- EUS-directed transenteric ERCP (EDEE) is a novel, but nonetheless relatively safe and effective procedure to establish bile and pancreatic duct access in patients with SAA who are not candidates for other drainage modalities.
- AEs occur in 3% to 5% of cases and can be minimized with careful preprocedure planning.

 Video content accompanies this article at http://www.giendo.theclinics.com.

INTRODUCTION

Patients with pancreaticobiliary disease and surgically altered anatomy (SAA) pose a unique challenge for the practicing endoscopist. Traditional pancreaticobiliary access in such patients has required either device-assisted endoscopic retrograde cholangiopancreatography (DAE) or percutaneous transhepatic biliary drainage (PTBD) owing to the length of the small intestine that must first be traversed. Limitations to DAE include suboptimal success rates and a lack of dedicated ERCP accessories to perform therapeutic maneuvers, resulting in modest diagnostic and therapeutic success rates of

[a] Division of Gastroenterology and Hepatology, Weill Cornell Medicine, 1283 York Avenue, 9th Floor, New York, NY 10065, USA; [b] Division of Gastroenterology and Hepatology, Mayo Clinic, 200 1st Street Southwest, Rochester, MN 55905, USA
* Corresponding author.
E-mail address: mah4040@med.cornell.edu
Twitter: @MarkHanscomMD (M.H.)

Gastrointest Endoscopy Clin N Am 34 (2024) 511–522
https://doi.org/10.1016/j.giec.2024.02.006
1052-5157/24/© 2024 Elsevier Inc. All rights reserved.

69.4% and 61%, respectively. In addition, adverse events (AEs) can occur in up to 6.5% of cases, including serious AEs such as pancreatitis (2.2%), bleeding (0.4%), and perforation (0.8%).[1] PTBD is more effective but likewise carries a high risk of AEs reaching up to 60%, including catheter occlusion, catheter dislodgement, and infection, with a resultant high rate of hospital readmissions.[2,3]

The introduction of several new endoscopic stents, including an electrocautery enhanced lumen apposing metal stent (ECE-LAMS) (AXIOS, Boston Scientific, Marlborough, MA) and a nonforeshortening, covered metal stent (VIABIL, GORE Medical, Flagstaff, AZ) has led to the emergence of endoscopic ultrasound-guided biliary drainage (EUS-BD). EUS-BD, which comprises the rendezvous technique, antegrade drainage, and transluminal drainage, has been demonstrated to be safe and effective, with excellent technical (95%) and clinical (92%) success rates, but at the expense of an increased rate of AEs, which can surpass 23%.[4] Similar to with DAE, EUS-BD is also disadvantaged by a lack of dedicated accessories and therapeutic maneuvers.

Building upon the success of EUS-BD, several authors have also described a technique termed EUS-directed transenteric ERCP (EDEE), which entails the creation of a transgastric or transenteric anastomosis between the proximal gastrointestinal tract and a loop of distal small bowel containing the biliary orifice.[5] Following anastomosis creation using a LAMS, an endoscope can be advanced through the stent in order to bypass the intervening small bowel and access the papilla in a more standard retrograde fashion and with the full suite of ERCP accessories available. Perhaps the most well-known example of EDEE is the EUS-directed transgastric ERCP (EDGE) procedure, in which a new connection is formed between the gastric pouch and remnant stomach in patients with RYGB anatomy, which will be discussed elsewhere. Here, we will focus on transenteric ERCP in patients with non-RYGB SAA in order to facilitate access to the papilla or bilioenteric anastomosis.

SURGICALLY ALTERED ANATOMY

EDEE has been performed across multiple forms of SAA. The most common postsurgical anatomy encountered with EDEE is that of the Roux-en-Y hepaticojejunostomy (RYHJ) and Whipple procedure. Less often, EDEE with Billroth II and duodenal switch anatomy have been described.[5,6]

Roux-en-Y Hepaticojejunostomy

Similar to RYGB, access to the biliary tree in RYHJ is challenging and at times not possible depending on the length of the roux limb. RYHJ is most often performed during deceased donor liver transplantation (DDLT), but it can also be seen in certain cases of bile duct injury repair following cholecystectomy, and with bile duct tumor resection. It requires the creation of a bilioenteric anastomosis, in which the remaining nonresected bile duct is fashioned to a loop of jejunum (the biliopancreatic limb) that is in turn anastomosed to the downstream small bowel through a jejunojejunostomy. DAE is successful in 79% of cases, but can be limited by an excessive length of the Roux or biliopancreatic limb, angulation of the jejunojejunal anastomosis, or postoperative adhesions.[7] Preprocedural planning is critical, and operative notes should be reviewed to elucidate the length of Roux and biliopancreatic limbs prior to embarking on endoscopic exploration. EDEE must account for the length of the biliopancreatic limb, as well, so as not to position the anastomosis too far downstream. The presence of a single or dual post-transplant biliary anastomosis should also be clarified.

Whipple Procedure (Pancreaticoduodenectomy)

Indications for a Whipple procedure include treating cancer at the pancreatic head, distal common bile duct, ampulla, and periampullary duodenum. In a classic Whipple procedure, the pancreatic head, distal stomach, duodenum, proximal jejunum, distal common bile duct, and gallbladder are resected. Postsurgical anatomy includes a gastrojejunostomy, with a biliopancreatic afferent limb that contains the choledocho- and pancreatico-jejunal anastomoses, and a separate efferent limb that leads to the downstream small bowel and colon. Pylorus-preserving Whipple procedures can also be encountered. Success of DAE, using a pediatric colonoscope or dedicated enteroscope, ranges from 82% to 88%.[7-9] In cases where EDEE is pursued, preprocedure planning is critical. The biliopancreatic limb must be distinguished from the efferent limb, and the location of the biliary anastomosis must be identified. Optimal positioning of the transenteric anastomosis is several centimeters downstream from the anastomosis, such that an endoscope can be advanced to the anastomosis in a straightforward and neutral position.

Billroth II

The Billroth II procedure includes a partial, distal gastrectomy with an end-to-side anastomosis between the remaining stomach and proximal jejunum. The papilla is located along the afferent jejunal limb, whereas the efferent limb leads to the distal small bowel and colon. Billroth II is encountered less frequently than in the past but can still be seen following surgical treatment for gastric cancer or complicated peptic ulcer disease. Depending on the length of the afferent limb, the papilla can often be reached with a duodenoscope or gastroscope, albeit with an increased rate of bowel perforation.[10] Thus, consideration is often given to alternative techniques. If EDEE is pursued, as with the Whipple procedure, the transenteric anastomosis should be placed several centimeters downstream to the papilla, such that the advancement of the endoscope through the fistula allows the papilla to be viewed *en face* and not from behind (terminus side).

PRE-PROCEDURE PLANNING

In general, EDEE is reserved for cases that have failed ERCP, DAE, and/or EUS-BD. Indications for EDEE include failed biliary cannulation, long post-surgical small bowel limbs, complex biliary pathology, and partial afferent limb obstruction precluding traditional endoscopic access.[11] EDEE can be of particular benefit when the patient prefers to avoid percutaneous drainage, and EUS-BD is either not possible (eg, because of an absence of bile duct dilation), or not well suited to managing the pathology at hand, (eg, such as with distal common bile duct disease requiring repeat interventions and expanded therapeutic accessories, such as electrohydraulic lithotripsy (EHL)). EDEE should also be considered when EUS-guided anastomosis creation is being entertained for other reasons, such as with EUS-guided gastrojejunostomy (EUS-GJ) for the palliation of malignant gastric outlet obstruction (GOO). For example, in cases of obstructing pancreatic head cancer, a well-placed gastrojejunostomy, in the 3rd or 4th portion of the duodenum, can both alleviate the patient's GOO and allow for future access to the papilla retrograde through the stent.

To maximize success with EDEE and to minimize potential AEs, a preprocedure checklist can be helpful (**Table 1**). Informed consent should be obtained in all cases, including a specific discussion of the alternative endoscopic and percutaneous options. Surgical consultation is also encouraged, in particular if the patient is or might become a candidate for resection. Labs should be reviewed, and coagulopathies

Table 1
Preprocedure checklist prior to EDEE

Step	Details
Informed consent	Including a discussion of the risks and benefits, as well as alternative options such as percutaneous drainage and other endoscopic modalities.
Surgical consultation	To ensure EDEE does not disqualify a patient from surgical candidacy.
Review labs	In general, EDEE is considered safe with platelets >50,000 and INR <2.0.
Review imaging	Contrast-enhanced cross-sectional imaging is helpful to (i) define the anatomy, (ii) plan the route of transenteric anastomosis, and (iii) evaluate for potential complications (eg, ascites, intervening bowel).
Review operative notes	Specific answers to seek out include (i) what is the postsurgical anatomy, (ii) how long is the Roux and/or bilioenteric limb, and (iii) is there a single or dual anastomosis (with RYHJ)?
Plan procedural approach	Decide how the bilioenteric limb will be accessed and distended. In addition, decide whether single-session or staged EDEE will be pursued.
Collect needed equipment	Possible equipment list includes: therapeutic gastroscope, linear echoendoscope, 19 gauge fine-needle aspiration needle, 0.025 inch guidewire, saline/contrast/methylene blue mixture, 15 or 20 mm ECE-LAMS, TTS balloon dilator, sphincterotome, plastic, and fully covered metal biliary stents.
Plan for adverse events	Including the collection of needed equipment to salvage perforation or stent migration (eg, guidewire, retrieval forceps, TTS FCSEMS).

corrected. Like other forms of interventional EUS, EDEE is considered a high risk procedure and antithrombotic agents should be held as appropriate.[12]

It is important to have a plan of approach prior to attempting EDEE. The goal is to obtain the shortest and least angulated route to the ampulla or anastomosis, such that future attempts at cannulation are made simple. Preprocedure imaging should be reviewed, with attention to the location of the anticipated transenteric anastomosis and its relation to the biliary orifice. Operative notes should also be reviewed in detail. In patients with a hepaticojejunostomy, whether there is a single or dual anastomosis (separate left and right anastomoses) should be clarified.

Lastly, all needed equipment should be made available, including what would be needed for endoscopic rescue in the case of AEs (**Table 2**). The performing endoscopist should be comfortable managing adverse events (AEs) and well-versed in salvage endoscopic techniques.

PROCEDURAL APPROACH

Several methods have been described for EDEE, with most variations occurring during the identification and distension of the biliopancreatic limb step. Our procedural approach is as follows (Video 1).

- Locate the biliopancreatic limb. In most cases, we first perform an upper endoscopy to better evaluate the patient's postsurgical anatomy and attempt to locate the biliopancreatic limb. In cases whereby the biliopancreatic limb can be reached endoscopically, our preference is to then advance a wire-guided 7

Table 2
Partial equipment list and procedural uses

Equipment	Procedural Uses
Echoendoscope	Linear echoendoscope, ± a therapeutic gastroscope to first locate and distend the biliopancreatic limb.
Nasobiliary catheter	Either a 7 Fr or 8.5 Fr catheter, used to instill contrast mixture and distend the bilioenteric limb.
EUS needle	19-gauge fine needle aspiration needle, if needed to confirm or distend the target bowel.
Percutaneous biliary drain	When present, can be used to locate and distend the target bowel. Pre-existing PTD should be exchanged for one without side holes to prevent bile duct injury.
Contrast/saline mixture	We favor a saline/contrast mixture, with a few drops of methylene blue for color. Saline is preferred over sterile water, due to the risk of water intoxication and electrolyte disturbances with the latter.
ECE-LAMS	Either a 15- or 20-mm LAMS depending on patient's anatomy and plan of approach.
Guidewires	0.025-inch hydrophilic guidewire, to be used with cold LAMS placement or if stent dilation or rescue maneuvers are needed.
Balloon dilator	Through-the-scope (TTS) balloon dilator, based on the size of the stent, to expand the deployed LAMS if needed.
Fully covered self-expandable metal stent (FCSEMS)	Such as a covered esophageal stent, or one with antimigration fins, to rescue a migrated or misdeployed LAMS.
Fluoroscopy	To help locate the bilioenteric limb, deploy the LAMS, and perform ERCP.

French nasobiliary catheter through the channel of a therapeutic gastroscope and into the biliopancreatic limb for subsequent fluid distension. Exceptions are made in the case of a previously placed percutaneous transhepatic drain (PTD), which is used instead for identification and distension of the target loop of bowel.

- Distend the biliopancreatic limb. The gastroscope is then removed and a linear echoendoscope is advanced into the stomach. A mixture of dilute contrast

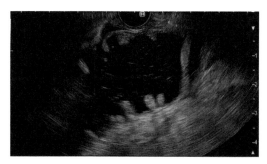

Fig. 1. Endosonographic view of the target loop of bowel being distended. Echogenic bubbles can be seen, confirming the identification of the bilioenteric limb as it fills with fluid.

and methylene blue is instilled through the nasobiliary catheter to distend the target bowel **(Fig. 1)**. Glucagon (2 mg, IV, push bolus) is administered to halt small bowel peristalsis.

- Confirm the target small bowel under EUS. The distended small bowel is targeted endosonographically. If a PTD or a nasobiliary catheter was placed, this serves as an additional marker. Color doppler ultrasound (US) is used to identify intervening vessels. The distance between the 2 luminal walls is measured and should be < 10 mm to proceed. Fluoroscopy should be used liberally when identifying a target limb, taking note of the endoscope's position, rotation, and distance to the biliary anastomosis. Choosing a puncture site that allows the echoendoscope to maintain a neutral, straight position will help with stent deployment and subsequent ERCP **(Fig. 2)**.
- (Optional) Puncture of target bowel. In cases whereby direct puncture and distension of the target bowel is needed, or further confirmation of the target bowel is required, the target bowel can be first punctured using a 19 gauge "finder" needle. Aspiration of blue-tinged fluid confirms appropriate positioning. The needle is then withdrawn, and the procedure continued.
- Placement of ECE-LAMS. The ECE-LAMS is advanced into position and cautery is applied. The target bowel is accessed and the stent is deployed, starting with the release of the proximal flange under endosonographic and fluoroscopic vision. Finally, the distal flange is released under endoscopic and fluoroscopic vision **(Figs. 3 and 4)**. Positioning is confirmed with rapid drainage of blue effluent and visualization of small bowel mucosa beyond the proximal flange of the LAMS. Frequently, the nasobiliary catheter can also be visualized through the lumen of the LAMS postdeployment.
- (Optional) Dilate the LAMS. If further confirmation of stent positioning is wanted, or is single-session EDEE is pursued, the stent can be dilated. First, a 0.025-inch angled hydrophilic guidewire is advanced beyond the stent and coiled in the small bowel. Then, a dilating balloon is advanced over the guidewire and inflated to open the stent **(Fig. 5)**.
- Perform ERCP. If single-session EDEE is indicated, the echoendoscope is exchanged for a gastroscope or duodenoscope, which is advanced through the LAMS into the target small bowel and ERCP is performed. If staged EDEE

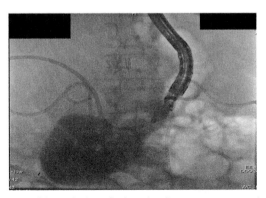

Fig. 2. The target loop of bowel identified under fluoroscopy. Note the straight, neutral positioning of the echoendoscope, which will facilitate ease of stent deployment and subsequent traversal.

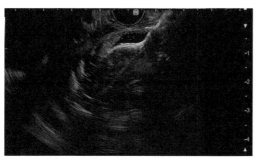

Fig. 3. The bilioenteric limb is accessed using the ECE-LAMS, with deployment of the first flange of the stent under endosonographic vision.

is indicated, the procedure is ended and the patient then returns after 3 to 4 weeks for the ERCP portion.

Multiple variations on the above procedural steps exist.[6,11] If the biliopancreatic limb can be reached with an endoscope, the dilute contrast with methylene blue mixture can be instilled directly through the therapeutic channel of the endoscope to distend the target bowel. Glucagon is administered to halt peristalsis, and the endoscope can be quickly exchanged for the echoendoscope, and steps #3 to 5 continued. Alternatively, if a nasobiliary drain is not available, other endoscopic accessories (eg, balloon catheter, tapered cannula) can also be used to instill the contrast and methylene blue mixture. If a PTD has been previously placed, the drain can be used to both locate the target small bowel and instill the contrast mixture. When using a PTD, it should first be exchanged for a tube with side holes only on the locking loop (Mac-Loc, Cook Medical, Winston-Salem, NC) to prevent overdistension of the intrahepatic bile ducts, which can lead to bile duct injury and bile leak. In cases of afferent limb syndrome, the target limb of small bowel is often markedly dilated, making for easier recognition and targeting under EUS. Lastly, direct EUS-guided puncture of the

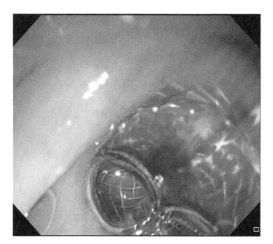

Fig. 4. The second flange of the LAMS is then deployed in the gastrointestinal tract lumen under endoscopic and fluoroscopic vision, with rapid return of blue-tinged effluent confirming appropriate transenteric positioning.

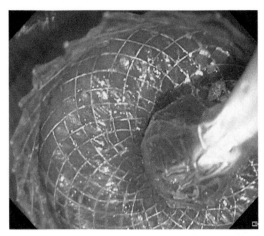

Fig. 5. If same-session EDEE is indicated, or visualization of the distal small bowel mucosa is wanted to confirm positioning, the LAMS can be dilated using a TTS dilating balloon. Here, a 10 mm biliary dilating balloon (Hurricane, Boston Scientific, Marlborough, MA) is used to dilate the stent.

biliopancreatic limb is an alternative option to distend the small bowel. In this technique, the small bowel is punctured with a 19-gauge needle, through which the contrast mixture is instilled to distend the limb. Opacification of the biliopancreatic limb, and sometimes the distal bile duct, confirms correct positioning. The needle can then be removed, and stent placement pursued of the newly distended small bowel.

Both ECE-LAMS (hot) placement and non-ECE (cold) LAMS placement have been described, although the authors favor the former. In the latter technique, the stent is advanced over an 0.025-inch or 0.035-inch guidewire that is first coiled in the target bowel under fluoroscopy. The size of the selected stent selected depends on procedural factors, including whether single-session ERCP is anticipated, the site of the anastomosis (transgastric vs transenteric), and the diameter of the distended target bowel. For most cases, we find that a 15 mm ECE-LAMS suffices.

Once the stent is in place, an endoscope can then be advanced through the new anastomosis and into bilioenteric limb (**Fig. 6**). Either a gastroscope with a clear cap or a duodenoscope can be used, depending on the postsurgical anatomy and what will best facilitate the approach to the biliary orifice. The upstream and downstream limb can appear similar endoscopically, and fluoroscopy is helpful to ascertain the correct direction. If same-session ERCP is pursued, the use of endoscopic suturing or silicon lubrication applied to the endoscope can facilitate stent traversal and reduce the risk of stent migration. Once the biliary orifice is identified, ERCP can be performed according to standard practice.

RECOVERY AND REHABILITATION

Postprocedure recovery and rehabilitation is often short, barring AEs. Patients can be started on a liquid diet on the same day as the procedure, followed by rapid advancement to a stent-based diet while the stent remains *in situ*. Mean hospital duration following the procedure ranges from 1 to 4.7 days.[5,6] In our experience, expedited same day or next day discharge can also be considered if the patient recovers well with no signs of AEs.

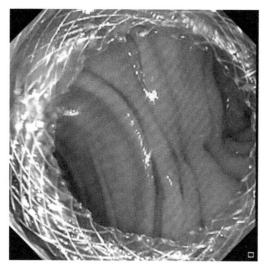

Fig. 6. Following deployment, the endoscope can be advanced into the target loop of small bowel containing the biliary orifice. The upstream and downstream limb can appear similar, and fluoroscopy is helpful in determining the correct approach.

Overall, periprocedural AEs range from 3% to 6%, and overall AEs from 18% to 28%.[5,6] In a retrospective review of 18 patients who underwent EDEE, 1 patient experienced immediate postprocedural abdominal pain that was managed conservatively. Four additional patients required endoscopic reintervention because of stent occlusion.[11] In a separate review of 32 patients post-EDEE, 1 patient experienced moderate but self-limited bleeding, and 5 patients experienced late AEs comprising of 4 cases of stent migration and 1 case of a persistent biliocutaneous fistula in a patient who had a PTD.[6]

The most feared AE of EDEE is acute stent dislodgement or perforation.[13] Stent migration can be minimized by performing a staged EDEE, with the ERCP component occurring a minimum of 3 to 4 weeks following LAMS placement once the anastomosis has matured. If single session EDEE is pursued, strong consideration should be given to using a large caliber LAMS (eg, 20 mm) and suturing the stent in place prior to traversal with the endoscope. Additionally, the use of a small caliber, diagnostic duodenoscope, if available may also mitigate the risk of stent dislodgement. Upon withdrawing the scope after ERCP, leaving a trailing guidewire behind allows for luminal access should the stent become dislodged for salvage stent placement.

In the acute setting, the early recognition of stent dislodgement is critical, as it is equivalent to perforation. Once recognized, salvage maneuvers can be performed to rescue the dislodged stent, including repeat stenting if a guidewire has been maintained or a stent-in-stent technique, in which an FCSEMS is placed in coaxial fashion within the LAMS to better bridge the anastomosis. Late migration after tract maturation can be treated with simple stent replacement.

MANAGEMENT

Following successful EDEE, several questions must be addressed. First, the endoscopist must decide whether to perform single-session or staged EDEE. If single-session ERCP is planned, consideration should also be given to suturing the LAMS in place, to reduce the chance of dislodgement. In our practice, we prefer to perform staged EDEE whenever possible, to minimize the risk of stent migration, particularly when creating a small bowel-to-small bowel anastomosis. To this end, we favor the use of a 15 mm ECE-LAMS with second stage EDEE after 3 to 4 weeks to allow for complete tract maturation.

Second, the endoscopist must decide whether repeated access to the major papilla is indicated after EDEE. If so, the anastomosis must be maintained to prevent spontaneous closure. This is possible with either repeated exchange of the LAMS (to prevent the delamination of the silicone coating and tissue ingrowth) or exchange of the LAMS for double pigtail plastic stents. Our practice is to schedule a repeat EGD 3 to 6 months from the EDEE, with either removal or exchange of the LAMS for plastic stents at that time depending on the anticipated need for repeat access to the bile duct. Once access to the bile duct is no longer needed, the prostheses can be removed, and the fistula allowed to spontaneously close.

If a PTD has been placed, this can often be removed at the end of the EDEE, provided that enough time has passed from its placement to allow for tract maturation and adequate internal drainage has been established during the EDEE. Close collaboration with Interventional Radiology is encouraged.

OUTCOMES

Few studies have been published on the outcomes of EDEE, but those that have appear promising. In the largest report to date, Mutignani and colleagues described EDEE in 32 patients with either RYHJ or Whipple anatomy. Indications included anastomotic stricture (69%), bile duct stricture (12.5%), previous stent entrapment (9.4%), choledocholithiasis (6.25%), and biliary fistula (3%). Technical success was 96.9%, with 1 technical failure occurring because of an inability to achieve optimal positioning of the echoendoscope. There was 1 periprocedural AE that was moderate in severity (self-limited bleeding).[6]

Khashab and colleagues performed a multicenter, retrospective review comprising 7 hospitals and 18 total patients. The most common indications for EDEE were malignant biliary stricture (44.4%), biliary stones (27.8%), benign biliary stricture (22.2%), and retained pancreatic stent resulting in recurrent pancreatitis (5.6%). The most common postsurgical anatomy encountered was Whipple procedure (55.5%), RYHJ (33.3%), Billroth II (5.6%), and duodenal switch (5.6%). EDEE was of technical and clinical success in 17/18 (94.4%) patients, with the sole case of technical and clinical failure occurring because of a luminal stricture distal to the gastrojejunostomy that precluded passage of the duodenoscope. AEs occurred in 5.6% of patients, consisting of 1 case of abdominal pain that was managed conservatively. No late AEs were reported.[5]

Storm and colleagues reported EDEE using a 15 mm ECE-LAMS in a patient with RYHJ and anastomotic stricture. The case required stent rescue using a 10 mm × 6 cm covered metal stent with antimigration fins, highlighting the importance of preprocedural planning.

Delayed follow-up between 34 and 88 days has been reported, and while late AEs appear uncommon, repeat interventions for migrated and/or occluded stents are not infrequent, and are needed in 18% to 28% of patients.[5,6,14]

SUMMARY

Patients with SAA are being frequently encountered in clinical practice, owing to the rising rates of bariatric surgeries and liver transplantation.[15–17] Endoscopic management of pancreaticobiliary disease, as with traditional ERCP, is more challenging in patients with SAA because of the uncertainty of reaching the biliary orifice and limited accessories to accomplish therapeutic maneuvers once in position. DAE is associated with suboptimal success rates, and PTBD, while effective, is associated with a high rate of AEs, poor patient tolerance, and need for repeat intervention. EUS-BD is an attractive option in certain patients, but not all patients are candidates for EUS-BD.

EDEE is a relatively safe and effective option for the management of pancreaticobiliary disease in patients with SAA who have failed or are otherwise not candidates for traditional ERCP. Compared with alternative techniques, EDEE allows for complete endoscopic access to the biliary tree, with the use of the full suite of ERCP accessories. Furthermore, EDEE allows for repeated access to the ampullary and pancreaticobiliary region in patients with distal or complex pathology. EDEE is particularly useful in several scenarios: (i) inability to perform EUS-BD because of decompressed or inaccessible bile ducts, (ii) need for access to the distal bile ducts or periampullary/pancreaticobiliary region (eg, for the EUS examination of suspected ampullary tumor), and (iii) when EUS-guided anastomosis (eg, EUS-GJ) is being concurrently pursued for lumenal obstruction.

EDEE remains a relatively novel procedure, with few, small, published studies. EDEE is considered technically challenging and should be performed by experts in referral centers with multidisciplinary support. Preprocedure planning is critical to ensuring an optimal outcome. AEs are uncommon, but can be severe, and performing endoscopists should be comfortable recognizing and managing them in the peri and postprocedural setting.

CLINICS CARE POINTS

- EDEE is a relatively safe and effective alternative for the management of pancreaticobiliary disease in patients with SAA who are either not candidates for or have failed alternative techniques for biliary drainage.
- EDEE can be of particular benefit in appropriate candidates who need repeated access to the distal biliary tree or periampullary region, who lack dilated bile ducts to allow for EUS-BD, or who are undergoing EUS-anastomosis for concurrent reasons.
- Preprocedural planning is critical, and special emphasis should be placed on how the endoscopist plans to access and dilate the target limb of small bowel.
- In cases whereby a PTBD is used to instill fluid, one should first exchange the drain for one without intraductal side holes to prevent bile duct blow out and resultant bile leak.
- If long term access to the biliary orifice is required, consider leaving plastic stents in the transenteric anastomosis to maintain patency.

DISCLOSURE

R. Law is a consultant for ConMed and Medtronic and receives royalties from UpToDate.

SUPPLEMENTARY DATA

Supplementary data to this article can be found online at https://doi.org/10.1016/j.giec.2024.02.006.

REFERENCES

1. Inamdar S, Slattery E, Sejpal DV, et al. Systematic review and meta-analysis of single-balloon enteroscopy–assisted ERCP in patients with surgically altered GI anatomy. Gastrointest Endosc 2015;82(1):9–19.
2. Sarwar A, Hostage CA, Weinstein JL, et al. Causes and rates of 30-day readmissions after percutaneous transhepatic biliary drainage procedure. Radiology 2019;290(3):722–9.
3. Nennstiel S, Weber A, Frick G, et al. Drainage-related complications in percutaneous transhepatic biliary drainage: an analysis over 10 years. J Clin Gastroenterol 2015;49(9):764–70.
4. Wang K, Zhu J, Xing L, et al. Assessment of efficacy and safety of EUS-guided biliary drainage: a systematic review. Gastrointest Endosc 2016;83(6):1218–27.
5. Ichkhanian Y, Yang J, James TW, et al. EUS-directed transenteric ERCP in non-Roux-en-Y gastric bypass surgical anatomy patients (with video). Gastrointest Endosc 2020;91(5):1188–94.e2.
6. Mutignani M, Bonato G, Dioscoridi L, et al. EUS-guided enteroenteral bypass for transenteric ERCP: building on prior knowledge. Gastrointest Endosc 2021; 93(1):279.
7. Itokawa F, Itoi T, Ishii K, et al. Single- and double-balloon enteroscopy-assisted endoscopic retrograde cholangiopancreatography in patients with R oux-en- Y plus hepaticojejunostomy anastomosis and W hipple resection. Dig Endosc 2014;26(S2):136–43.
8. Chahal P, Baron T, Topazian M, et al. Endoscopic retrograde cholangiopancreatography in post-Whipple patients. Endoscopy 2006;38(12):1241–5.
9. Li K, Huang YH, Yao W, et al. Adult colonoscopy or single-balloon enteroscopy-assisted ERCP in long-limb surgical bypass patients. Clin Res Hepatol Gastroenterol 2014;38(4):513–9.
10. Takano S, Fukasawa M, Shindo H, et al. Risk factors for perforation during endoscopic retrograde cholangiopancreatography in post-reconstruction intestinal tract. World J Clin Cases 2019;7(1):10–8.
11. Khashab MA. Endoscopic ultrasound-directed transenteric ERCP (EDEE) in patients with postsurgical anatomy – novel but challenging: Referring to Mutignani M et al. p. 1146–1150. Endoscopy 2019;51(12):1119–20.
12. Acosta RD, Abraham NS, Chandrasekhara V, et al. The management of antithrombotic agents for patients undergoing GI endoscopy. Gastrointest Endosc 2016;83(1):3–16.
13. Ghandour B, Bejjani M, Irani SS, et al. Classification, outcomes, and management of misdeployed stents during EUS-guided gastroenterostomy. Gastrointest Endosc 2022;95(1):80–9.
14. Chin J, Storm AC. Endoscopic ultrasound-guided gastrojejunostomy and rescue technique to simplify endoscopic retrograde cholangiopancreatography in surgically altered anatomy. ACG Case Rep J 2020;7(11):e00482.
15. Kwong AJ, Ebel NH, Kim WR, et al. OPTN/SRTR 2020 annual data report: liver. Am J Transplant 2022;22:204–309.
16. Terrault NA, Francoz C, Berenguer M, et al. Liver transplantation 2023: status report, current and future challenges. Clin Gastroenterol Hepatol 2023;21(8): 2150–66.
17. Overweight & obesity statistics | NIDDK. national institute of diabetes and digestive and kidney diseases. Available at: https://www.niddk.nih.gov/health-information/health-statistics/overweight-obesity. [Accessed 11 January 2023].

Endoscopic Ultrasonography-Guided Gallbladder Drainage

Shannon Melissa Chan, MBChB, FRCSEd, FHKAM (Surgery),
Anthony Yuen Bun Teoh, MBChB, FRCSEd, FHKAM (Surgery)*

KEYWORDS

- EUS-guided gallbladder drainage • EUS-GBD • Acute cholecystitis

KEY POINTS

- Indications, preoperative preparation of endoscopic ultrasound-guided gallbladder drainage (EUS-GBD).
- Approaches to EUS-GBD.
- Long-term management of lumen-apposing stent after EUS-GBD.
- Evidence of outcomes of EUS-GBD, as compared to other drainage options such as percutaneous gallbladder drainage and endoscopic transpapillary gallbladder drainage.
- A video of the needle first puncture approach accompanies this review article.

 Video content accompanies this article at http://www.giendo.theclinics.com.

INTRODUCTION

Acute cholecystitis is a common surgical condition with 50% to 70% of the cases occurring in the elderly.[1] Gallstones obstructing the flow of bile account for 90% of cases of cholecystitis, and is called calculous cholecystitis.[2] The blockage of bile flow leads to thickening and buildup of bile causing a distended and tense gallbladder. The gallbladder is initially sterile, but with obstruction often becomes subsequently infected by bacteria.[3] According to the Tokyo guidelines of 2018, the gold standard for management of cholecystitis in surgically fit patients is laparoscopic cholecystectomy (LC). LC is associated with a low risk of operative morbidity and mortality.[4,5] However, in elderly patients or patients with significant comorbidities, emergency LC can be associated with significant risk of morbidities (up to 41%) and mortalities (up to 19%).[6,7] Thus, in these patients several management options can be offered

Department of Surgery, Prince of Wales Hospital, The Chinese University of Hong Kong, Shatin, Hong Kong, China
* Corresponding author.
E-mail address: anthonyteoh@surgery.cuhk.edu.hk

Gastrointest Endoscopy Clin N Am 34 (2024) 523–535
https://doi.org/10.1016/j.giec.2024.02.010
1052-5157/24/© 2024 Elsevier Inc. All rights reserved.

including antibiotics alone, percutaneous cholecystostomy (percutaneous [PT]-gall-bladder drainage [GBD]), endoscopic transpapillary gallbladder drainage (ETP-GBD) or endoscopic ultrasound-guided gallbladder drainage (EUS-GBD).

HISTORY AND EVOLUTION

PT-GBD is the most established and frequently used technique for gallbladder drainage in high-risk patients.[7–10] However, complications including intrahepatic hemorrhage, pneumothorax, biliary peritonitis, and pneumonia have been reported in 6.2% of the patients (range 0%–25%). Furthermore, PT-GBD has several other disadvantages including risk of bile leakage, recurrent cholecystitis, inadvertent tube removal and migration (0%–25%), necessitating repeated procedures. The external catheter also induces discomfort, local pain, and cosmetic disfigurement.

ETP-GBD using a nasobiliary drain or plastic stents has been described since the 1990s[11] with the pooled technical success rate 80.9% and clinical response rate of 75.3%. The incidence of procedure-related adverse events (AEs) is 0% to 14%. The main limiting factor of this technique is the difficulty in cannulating the cystic duct, particularly in the presence of stone impacted at the Hartmann's pouch of the gallbladder or obstruction due to tumor or stent.

EUS-GBD in patients who are not fit for surgery has been described since 2007.[12–15] The technique uses EUS-guided creation of a cholecysto-gastric or duodenal fistula and placement of a stent for gallbladder drainage. It was initially described in 2007 with transmural placement of a 7Fr double pigtail stent into the gallbladder for a patient with unresectable hilar cholangiocarcinoma and acute cholecystitis.[13] The technique is an attractive alternative to PT-GBD or endoscopic transpapillary drainage of the gallbladder (ET-GBD) as it avoids the need to cannulate the cystic duct and obstructed stones, the need for the periodic exchange of stents, and lacks an external tube. The rapid advancement in stents available, notably a cautery-enhanced lumen-apposing stent (LAMS) has made the procedure safer and more reproducible. The flanges of these LAMS were designed to distribute pressure evenly and conform to the luminal wall (**Fig. 1**). They are also cautery-enhanced, thus allowing single-step placement, which decreases the need for the exchange of multiple instruments. The large luminal diameter stents also allow for access to the gallbladder for complete clearance of stones, and this may potentially reduce the risk of recurrent cholecystitis.[16]

Over the past few years, comparative trials, meta-analysis, randomized controlled trials and network meta-analysis have been published comparing the outcomes of these 3 drainage modalities. In the only randomized trial to date Teoh and colleagues

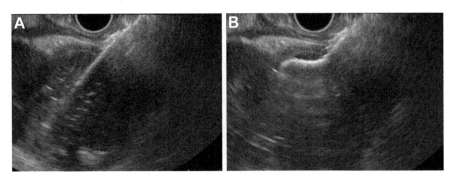

Fig. 1. (A) Direct puncture of the distended gallbladder with the cautery-enhanced LAMS and (B) distal flange being deployed.

showed that EUS-GBD achieved lower rates of reintervention and AEs at 1 year compared to PT-GBD.[17] These findings were also confirmed by subsequent meta-analyses.

INDICATIONS FOR ENDOSCOPIC ULTRASOUND-GUIDED GALLBLADDER DRAINAGE

The following are suggested indications for EUS-GBD (according to the most recent AGA guidelines)[18]:

1. Acute cholecystitis in surgically unfit patients[4]
2. Conversion (internalization) of indwelling cholecystostomy tubes when cholecystectomy is not planned[19]
3. Palliation of malignant biliary obstruction in patients who failed ERCP or EUS-GBD[20]

PATIENT SELECTION

According to current guidelines, EUS-GBD should be performed in patients who are at high risk for surgery as an alternative to PT-GBD.[4] If the procedure is offered to surgically fit patients, one would need to consider management issues that arise after creation of a cholecysto-duodenal or gastric fistula. A prospective case series did show that it is safe and feasible to perform cholecystectomy after EUS-GBD.[21] However, there is a theoretic risk of postoperative leakage particularly when repair of the fistula is required. Therefore it is crucial to obtain a consensus with the surgical team before placing a transmural gallbladder stent in a surgically fit patient.

Apart from the above indications, prophylactic EUS-GBD for patients at the time of self-expandable biliary metal stents placement for unresectable malignant biliary obstruction involving the cystic duct orifice has also been shown to decrease rate of acute cholecystitis (22.7% to 0%; $P = .049$).[22]

CONTRAINDICATIONS

Patients with perforated gallbladder, biliary peritonitis, massive ascites, and significant coagulopathy are contraindications to EUS-GBD. EUS-GBD appears to be safe in patients on anticoagulation, though it is recommended that these medications are withheld according to guidelines.[23] More data are needed in this area.

Preoperative/Pre-procedure Planning

Prep and patient positioning

Patients need to be fasted before the procedures per anesthesia guidelines. Antithrombotics should be withheld, if possible, per guidelines. Platelet and clotting profile should be checked and corrected as per guidelines. Broad spectrum intravenous antibiotics should be administered prior to the procedure.

This procedure can be performed either in the supine or prone position depending on endoscopists preference. The procedure can also be done entirely under EUS-guidance without fluoroscopy using a cautery-enhanced LAMS, and thus can also be done in a left lateral position.

Procedural approach

EUS-GBD can be performed with 2 methods depending on the stent availability and the anatomy. Cautery-enhanced LAMS is the best choice of stent to use as it avoids the cumbersome exchange of accessories during the procedure. Non-cautery enhanced LAMS or biliary covered self-expandable metal stents (CSEMS) can also be used. There are 2 main procedural approaches: (i) the direct puncture method and (ii) the conventional method.

i. Direct puncture method
   1. A suitable puncture site is first located in the gastric antrum or the duodenum. The gallbladder is punctured directly with the cautery equipped LAMS delivery system (see **Fig. 1**A).
   2. The distal flange is deployed under EUS guidance or fluoroscopic guidance (see **Fig. 1**B).
   3. Once the distal flange is deployed, the delivery system is pulled back with gentle tension to appose the two organs.
   4. The proximal flange can then be deployed with 2 methods: (i) endoscopic visualization and (ii) in-channel deployment. Endoscopic visualization was the method first described. With the AXIOS delivery system (Boston Scientific, Marlborough, MA, USA), a "black marker" would be visualized endoscopically upon right torque of the scope (**Fig. 2**A). Once the black mark is seen, the proximal flange can be deployed under endoscopic guidance. For the in-channel deployment method, the distal flange is deployed as usual with the endoscope tip pressed against the gastric or duodenal wall. The delivery system is then pulled back gently until a slight distortion of the distal stent flange within the gallbladder is seen on EUS view. The proximal stent flange is then completely deployed within the endoscope channel. The view is then changed to the luminal view, where a right torque and down scope position is applied to the endoscope. The stent should be visualized at the right upper corner of the endoscopic view (**Fig. 2**B). The stent is gradually pushed out of the channel by advancing the delivery system while maintaining a right torque force. The stent will be seen in the typical endoscopic view (**Fig. 2**C).

ii. Conventional approach (Video 1 shows the steps of this approach)
   1. After location of a suitable puncture site, the gallbladder is punctured with a 19G fine aspiration needle. Bile or pus is aspirated to confirm the position of the needle (**Fig. 3**), or contrast can be injected under fluoroscopic guidance.
   2. A 0.035 or 0.025 guidewire is inserted into the gallbladder to form a loop (**Fig. 4**).
   3. Exchange to a cautery-enhanced or regular LAMS. The LAMS is then deployed as described in the direct puncture approach.
   4. If a non-cautery-enhanced LAMS or CSEMS is used, the guidewire is exchanged to perform track dilation to allow the stent delivery system to pass into the gallbladder using a 4 mm dilating balloon with or without antecedent cautery with a 6Fr cystotome. Alternatively, a 7Fr rigid dilator (ES dilator, Zeon Medical Co., Tokyo, Japan) can also be used, if available.
   5. The LAMS is then deployed as described in direct puncture approach (**Figs. 5** and **6**).

In general, the direct puncture approach is preferred to avoid the cumbersome exchange of accessories and to shorten procedural time. However, the conventional approach is potentially safer, especially if the gallbladder is decompressed. The guidewire can potentially reduce risk of stent misdeployment and allows for salvage procedures such as insertion of additional stents if misdeployment occurs. This is especially useful when the gallbladder is suboptimally distended in cases of contracted gallbladder, or in situations for conversions to EUS-GBD after PT-GBD.

Puncture site: antrum or duodenum?
The puncture site for EUS-GBD can be in the gastric antrum or duodenum. However, according to a recent retrospective study with 3 year follow-up, drainage from the

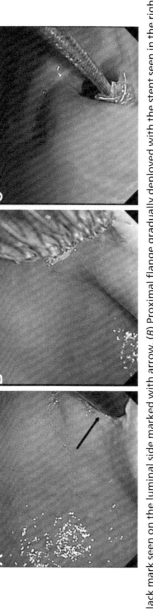

Fig. 2. (A) Black mark seen on the luminal side marked with arrow. (B) Proximal flange gradually deployed with the stent seen in the right upper corner. (C) Proximal flange fully deployed with pus drained.

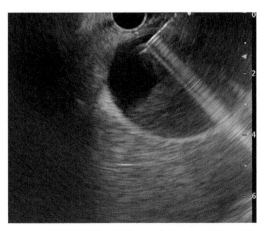

Fig. 3. Gallbladder was punctured with a 19G needle under EUS-guidance.

stomach was associated with significantly more late LAMS-related AEs in up to 37.5% of the patients (Martinez-Moreno EIO, in press). Furthermore, there are several factors also worth considering. Anatomically, the gallbladder is located closest to the first part of the duodenum. When the gallbladder is distended during acute cholecystitis, it can also be visualized at D1/2 or D2. The gallbladder can also be visualized from the antrum. However, the gastric antrum is located further away from the gallbladder. Drainage of the gallbladder from this site may cause tension and potentially increase the chance of buried stent syndrome and stent migration. Insertion of LAMS from the antrum theoretically also has a high risk of food reflux into the gallbladder with a resultant increased risk of recurrent cholecystitis, especially when large diameter metal stents are used. A third consideration is that whether the patient may become a candidate for cholecystectomy. Resecting a fistula to the antrum is easier than that to the duodenum. However, a comparative study did not show any significant difference in cholecystectomy completion between transgastric and transduodenal approaches.[21] A prospective randomized study is required to answer this question.

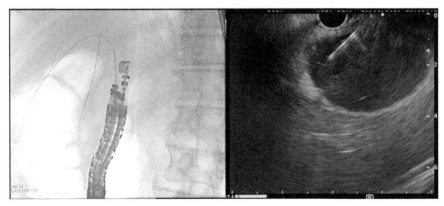

Fig. 4. After puncture of the gallbladder, a 0.025 guidewire was inserted to loop within the gallbladder.

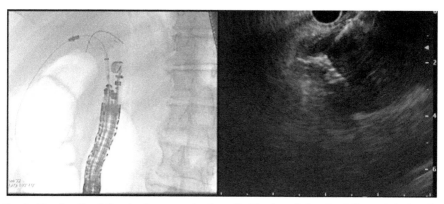

Fig. 5. The sheath of the stent was gradually pulled back and the distal flange is being deployed inside the gallbladder under EUS and fluoroscopy guidance.

Choice of stents

Metal stents are preferred over plastic stents in EUS-gallbladder drainage procedures.[24] Fully covered metal stents are recommended for transmural drainage procedure to prevent bile leakage between the gallbladder and the outer wall of the stomach or duodenum.[24] There are currently LAMS available from different companies. In general, the lumen diameters available include 6, 8, 10, 15, 16, and 20 mm. The most common interflange distance is 10 mm, but 15 and 20 mm lengths are also available. In general, the distance between the gastric/duodenal wall and the gallbladder wall should be less than 10 mm. Endoscopists must be wary of double puncture of the duodenal wall or puncture through pylorus in cases where the measured distance is greater than 10 mm.

The practice of plastic pigtail stent placement after LAMS insertion is also variable worldwide. Most endoscopists will insert a plastic pigtail in patients with larger stones

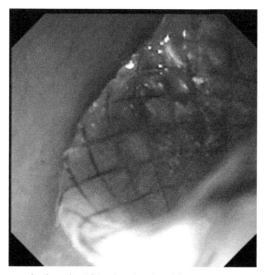

Fig. 6. Proximal flange deployed within the duodenal lumen.

to avoid stent occlusion by stones. Another potential benefit is to prevent the stent from impinging onto the back wall of the gallbladder, which may lead to intermittent stent obstruction or bleeding.

Postprocedural care
Patients can resume normal diet the day after the procedure if the sepsis is subsiding. This is evident with decrease in abdominal pain, improvement in peritoneal signs, and decrease in fever and inflammatory markers.

Long-term management
There is currently no consensus on long-term management of the gallstones and LAMS after EUS-GBD. Some centers perform cholecystoscopy 4 weeks later for stone clearance and stent removal. Some centers adopt a more conservative approach and leave the stent in place long-term, though the risks a permanent indwelling LAMS include stent erosion and stent migration.

Choi and colleagues reported a 7.1% AW rate in a median follow-up of 275 days after LAMS EUS-GBD. Two patients had asymptomatic distal stent migrations and 2 patients developed acute cholecystitis with stent occlusion. The cumulative stent patency rate was 86%.[25] Walter and colleagues also reported no AEs after a median follow-up of 364 days.[26] Stent erosion resulting in duodenal ulcer and upper gastrointestinal bleeding was also reported by Teoh and colleagues after 4 months of LAMS insertion.[27] Perez-Miranda and colleagues reported a 1 year cumulative risk of recurrent biliary events of 9.7% (4.1%–21.8%) and 1 year risk of AEs and of severe AEs of 18.8% (11%–31.2%) and 7.9% (3.3%–18.2%), respectively.[28] Therefore, it is the practice of some centers to remove the gallstones followed by stent removal. With the use of LAMS, a forward-viewing endoscope can be inserted via the stent into the gallbladder. This allows for a wide range of diagnostic and therapeutic procedures. Chan and colleagues reported a retrospective study of in 25 patients with 29 cholecystoscopies performed.[16] The overall technical success rate was 93.1%. The overall stone clearance rate was 88% after a mean (SD) number of 1.25 (0.46) sessions of cholecystoscopy. After stone clearance, the LAMS were removed with rat tooth forceps and a double pigtail was inserted to retain the fistula tract in case of future cholecystitis. With the above evidence, Ogura and colleagues suggested that perhaps permanent stent placement may be suitable for patients with shorter expected survival in order to avoid repeated endoscopic procedures. In patients with longer expected survival, stent removal may be more suitable to reduce stent-related complications.[29] There has been a case report on delamination of the LAMS with mucosa ingrowth after 15 months of placement for EUS-guided gastroenterotomy.[30] The authors hence suggested stent exchange in patients with survival of more than 12 months.

Still other endoscopists prefer to exchange the LAMS for 2 side-by-side plastic double pigtail stents that remain in place indefintely.[31]

Outcomes of endoscopic ultrasound-guided gallbladder drainage
Numerous studies have reported the outcomes of EUS-GBD for treatment of acute cholecystitis. In the majority of these studies, the gallbladder was drained by an EUS-specific stent with antimigratory properties.[32–35] A technical success of 90% to 98.7% and a clinical success of 89% to 98.4% were reported. AE rates were between 4.8% and 22% and included bleeding, recurrent cholecystitis, stent migration, pneumoperitoneum, and occlusion. Comparative studies are discussed in the following section.

Percutaneous cholecystostomy gallbladder drainage versus endoscopic ultrasound guided gallbladder drainage

Several comparative studies between EUS-GBD and PT-GBD were published.[32–35] The two procedures have similar technical (EUS-GBD vs PT-GBD = 85.7–96.6% vs 99%–100%) and clinical success rates (EUS-GBD vs PT-GBD = 89.8–95% vs 86%–94.9%).[32,33,35] PT-GBD was shown to be associated with more AEs and more unplanned admissions.[17,33] It was also shown to have a higher need for reintervention.[32] EUS-GBD is also associated with a significantly lower 1 year AEs rates ($P < .001$) and readmission rates ($P < .001$).[34] The majority of these were due to tube-related problems in the PT-GBD group. Irani and colleagues also reported lower postprocedural pain scores in the EUS-GBD group.[34] In a more recent randomized controlled trial, EUS-GBD was shown to be associated with a lower rate of recurrent cholecystitis at 1 year. Postprocedural pain scores and analgesic requirements were also less in the EUS-GBD group ($P = .034$).[17]

In addition, a meta-analysis that included 5 comparative studies (206 patients in the EUS-GBD group versus 289 patients in the PT-GBD group), concluded that EUS-GBD had fewer AEs than PT-GBD (odds ratio [OR] 0.43, 95% confidence interval [CI] 0.18–1.00; $P = .05$; I (2) = 66%), shorter hospital stays, with pooled standard mean difference of –2.53 (95 %CI - 4.28 to –0.78; $P = .005$; I (2) = 98%), and required significantly fewer reinterventions (OR 0.16, 95% CI 0.04–0.042; $P < .001$; I (2) = 32%) resulting in significantly fewer unplanned readmissions (OR 0.16, 95% CI 0.05–0.53; $P = .003$; I (2) = 79%).[10]

Endoscopic ultrasound guided gallbladder drainage versus endoscopic transpapillary gallbladder drainage

ET-GBD refers to the insertion of either a transpapillary double pigtail or a nasobiliary drain into the gallbladder. The procedure is technically demanding since the cystic duct is often torturous and contains valves, leading to difficult cannulation. Outcomes of this procedure varies widely. A systematic review revealed pooled success and AE rates of 96% and 6.3%, respectively.[11,36–39] Another meta-analysis comparing EUS-GBD versus ET-GBD for patients with high surgical risk with acute cholecystitis included 5 studies with a total of 857 (EUS-GBD vs ET-GBD: 259 vs 598 patients).[40] Compared to ET-GBD, EUS-GBD was associated with higher technical (pooled OR 5.22 [95% CI 2.03–13.44; $P = .0006$; $I^2 = 20\%$]) and clinical success rates (pooled OR 4.16 [95% CI 2.00–8.66; $P = .0001$; $I^2 = 19\%$]). In terms of overall AE rate, there was no difference (pooled OR 1.30 [95% CI 0.77–2.22; $P = .33$, $I^2 = 0\%$]). A more recent propensity score-matched analysis confirmed the above findings of high technical success with EUS-GBD.[41] The early AE rate did not differ significantly between the two methods (7.8% vs 8.9%, $P = 1.000$). The overall late AE rate was significantly lower with EUS-GBD (5.0% vs 16.4%, $P = .029$).

Endoscopic ultrasound guided gallbladder drainage versus percutaneous cholecystostomy gallbladder drainage versus endoscopic transpapillary gallbladder drainage

In the only study comparing these 3 arms in a systemic review and network analysis, 10 studies were included.[42] EUS-GBD had the lowest risk of recurrent cholecystitis compared with other modalities (relative risk [RR] for EUS-GBD vs PT-GBD vs ET-GBD, 1.089 vs 2.02 vs 2.891), whereas ET-GBD was associated with the lowest rates of mortality (RR for EUS-GBD vs PT-GBD vs ET-GBD, 2.62 vs 2.09 vs 1.29). PT-GBD has the highest probability of unplanned admissions and reintervention while ET-GBD has the lowest mortality.

SUMMARY

EUS-GBD is established for patients with high surgical risks. Other drainage options include PT-GBD and ET-GBD. The best approach for the patient should be tailor-made. Long-term management of LAMS is still controversial. More randomized trials and prospective data are required.

CLINICS CARE POINTS

- EUS-GBD is an established option for patients who suffer from acute calculous cholecystitis and are at high risk for surgery
- Alternatives include ET-GBD and PT-GBD. The best method of drainage depends on the anatomy, presence of ascites, evidence of perforation/gangrene, patient's future surgical candidacy, and availability of expertise.
- Long-term management of LAMS is still controversial. LAMS can be left in place long term, but with the potential for AEs. Cholecystoscopy can also be performed at 4 to 6 weeks after the drainage procedure for stone removal and subsequent stent removal when stones are cleared. Alternatively, the initial metal stent can be replaced with plastic stents after maturation of the transmural tract.

DISCLOSURE

Prof. A.Y.B. Teoh is a consultant for CMR surgical, Boston Scientific, Cook, Taewoong, Microtech and MI Tech Medical Corporations.

SUPPLEMENTARY DATA

Supplementary data to this article can be found online at https://doi.org/10.1016/j.giec.2024.02.010.

REFERENCES

1. Borzellino G, de Manzoni G, Ricci F, et al. Emergency cholecystostomy and subsequent cholecystectomy for acute gallstone cholecystitis in the elderly. Br J Surg 1999;86:1521–5.
2. Strasberg SM. Clinical practice. Acute calculous cholecystitis. N Engl J Med 2008;358:2804–11.
3. Greenberger NJ, PG. Chapter 311. Diseases of the gallbaldder and bile ducts. Longo DL, Fauci AS, Kasper DL, et al, editors. Harrison's Principles of Internal Medicine 18e.
4. Mori Y, Itoi T, Baron TH, et al. Tokyo Guidelines 2018: management strategies for gallbladder drainage in patients with acute cholecystitis (with videos). J Hepatobiliary Pancreat Sci 2018;25:87–95.
5. Mayumi T, Okamoto K, Takada T, et al. Tokyo Guidelines 2018: management bundles for acute cholangitis and cholecystitis. J Hepatobiliary Pancreat Sci 2018;25: 96–100.
6. Kirshtein B, Bayme M, Bolotin A, et al. Laparoscopic cholecystectomy for acute cholecystitis in the elderly: is it safe? Surg Laparosc Endosc Percutan Tech 2008; 18:334–9.
7. Kortram K, de Vries Reilingh TS, Wiezer MJ, et al. Percutaneous drainage for acute calculous cholecystitis. Surg Endosc 2011;25:3642–6.

8. Winbladh A, Gullstrand P, Svanvik J, et al. Systematic review of cholecystostomy as a treatment option in acute cholecystitis. HPB (Oxford) 2009;11:183–93.
9. Ahmed O, Rogers AC, Bolger JC, et al. Meta-analysis of outcomes of endoscopic ultrasound-guided gallbladder drainage versus percutaneous cholecystostomy for the management of acute cholecystitis. Surg Endosc 2018;32:1627–35.
10. Luk SW, Irani S, Krishnamoorthi R, et al. Endoscopic ultrasound-guided gallbladder drainage versus percutaneous cholecystostomy for high risk surgical patients with acute cholecystitis: a systematic review and meta-analysis. Endoscopy 2019;51(8):722–32.
11. Itoi T, Coelho-Prabhu N, Baron TH. Endoscopic gallbladder drainage for management of acute cholecystitis. Gastrointest Endosc 2010;71:1038–45.
12. Lee SS, Park DH, Hwang CY, et al. EUS-guided transmural cholecystostomy as rescue management for acute cholecystitis in elderly or high-risk patients: a prospective feasibility study. Gastrointest Endosc 2007;66:1008–12.
13. Baron TH, Topazian MD. Endoscopic transduodenal drainage of the gallbladder: implications for endoluminal treatment of gallbladder disease. Gastrointest Endosc 2007;65:735–7.
14. Jang JW, Lee SS, Park DH, et al. Feasibility and safety of EUS-guided transgastric/transduodenal gallbladder drainage with single-step placement of a modified covered self-expandable metal stent in patients unsuitable for cholecystectomy. Gastrointest Endosc 2011;74:176–81.
15. Song TJ, Lee SS, Park DH, et al. Preliminary report on a new hybrid metal stent for EUS-guided biliary drainage (with videos). Gastrointest Endosc 2014;80:707–11.
16. Chan SM, Teoh AYB, Yip HC, et al. Feasibility of per-oral cholecystoscopy and advanced gallbladder interventions after EUS-guided gallbladder stenting (with video). Gastrointest Endosc 2017;85:1225–32.
17. Teoh AYB, Kitano M, Itoi T, et al. Endosonography-guided gallbladder drainage versus percutaneous cholecystostomy in very high-risk surgical patients with acute cholecystitis: an international randomised multicentre controlled superiority trial (DRAC 1). Gut 2020;69:1085–91.
18. Irani SS, Sharzehi K, Siddiqui UD. AGA Clinical Practice Update on Role of EUS-Guided Gallbladder Drainage in Acute Cholecystitis: Commentary. Clin Gastroenterol Hepatol 2023;21:1141–7.
19. Law R, Grimm IS, Stavas JM, et al. Conversion of Percutaneous Cholecystostomy to Internal Transmural Gallbladder Drainage Using an Endoscopic Ultrasound-Guided, Lumen-Apposing Metal Stent. Clin Gastroenterol Hepatol 2016;14:476–80.
20. Mangiavillano B, Moon JH, Facciorusso A, et al. Endoscopic ultrasound-guided gallbladder drainage as a first approach for jaundice palliation in unresectable malignant distal biliary obstruction: Prospective study. Dig Endosc 2024;36(3):351–8.
21. Saumoy M, Tyberg A, Brown E, et al. Successful Cholecystectomy After Endoscopic Ultrasound Gallbladder Drainage Compared With Percutaneous Cholecystostomy, Can it Be Done? J Clin Gastroenterol 2019;53:231–5.
22. Robles-Medranda C, Oleas R, Puga-Tejada M, et al. Prophylactic EUS-guided gallbladder drainage prevents acute cholecystitis in patients with malignant biliary obstruction and cystic duct orifice involvement: a randomized trial (with video). Gastrointest Endosc 2023;97:445–53.
23. Vozzo CF, Simons-Linares CR, Abou Saleh M, et al. Safety of EUS-guided gallbladder drainage using a lumen-apposing metal stent in patients requiring anticoagulation. VideoGIE 2020;5:500–503 e1.

24. Teoh AYB, Dhir V, Kida M, et al. Consensus guidelines on the optimal management in interventional EUS procedures: results from the Asian EUS group RAND/UCLA expert panel. Gut 2018;67:1209–28.
25. Choi JH, Lee SS, Choi JH, et al. Long-term outcomes after endoscopic ultrasonography-guided gallbladder drainage for acute cholecystitis. Endoscopy 2014;46:656–61.
26. Walter D, Teoh AY, Itoi T, et al. EUS-guided gall bladder drainage with a lumen-apposing metal stent: a prospective long-term evaluation. Gut 2016;65:6–8.
27. Chan EOT, Chan SM, Yip HC, et al. Gastrointestinal bleeding after endoscopic ultrasound-guided gallbladder drainage. Endoscopy 2020;52:E249–50.
28. Bazaga S, García-Alonso FJ, Aparicio Tormo JR, et al. Endoscopic ultrasound-guided gallbladder drainage with long-term lumen-apposing metal stent indwell: 1-year results from a prospective nationwide observational study. J Gastroenterol Hepatol 2024;39(2):360–8.
29. Ogura T, Higuchi K. Endoscopic ultrasound-guided gallbladder drainage: Current status and future prospects. Dig Endosc 2019;31(Suppl 1):55–64.
30. Gilman AJ, Baron TH. Delamination of a lumen-apposing metal stent with tissue ingrowth and stent-in-stent removal. Gastrointest Endosc 2023;98:451–3.
31. Trieu JA, Gilman AJ, Hathorn K, Baron TH. Large Single-center Experience with Long-term Outcomes of EUS-guided Transmural Gallbladder Drainage. J Clin Gastroenterol 2023. https://doi.org/10.1097/MCG.0000000000001957.
32. Tyberg A, Saumoy M, Sequeiros EV, et al. EUS-guided Versus Percutaneous Gallbladder Drainage: Isn't It Time to Convert? J Clin Gastroenterol 2018;52:79–84.
33. Teoh AYB, Serna C, Penas I, et al. Endoscopic ultrasound-guided gallbladder drainage reduces adverse events compared with percutaneous cholecystostomy in patients who are unfit for cholecystectomy. Endoscopy 2017;49:130–8.
34. Irani S, Ngamruengphong S, Teoh A, et al. Similar Efficacies of Endoscopic Ultrasound Gallbladder Drainage With a Lumen-Apposing Metal Stent Versus Percutaneous Transhepatic Gallbladder Drainage for Acute Cholecystitis. Clin Gastroenterol Hepatol 2017;15:738–45.
35. Choi JH, Kim HW, Lee JC, et al. Percutaneous transhepatic versus EUS-guided gallbladder drainage for malignant cystic duct obstruction. Gastrointest Endosc 2017;85:357–64.
36. Hasan MK, Itoi T, Varadarajulu S. Endoscopic management of acute cholecystitis. Gastrointest Endosc Clin N Am 2013;23:453–9.
37. Itoi T, Sofuni A, Itokawa F, et al. Endoscopic transpapillary gallbladder drainage in patients with acute cholecystitis in whom percutaneous transhepatic approach is contraindicated or anatomically impossible (with video). Gastrointest Endosc 2008;68:455–60.
38. Kedia P, Sharaiha RZ, Kumta NA, et al. Endoscopic gallbladder drainage compared with percutaneous drainage. Gastrointest Endosc 2015;82:1031–6.
39. Khan MA, Atiq O, Kubiliun N, et al. Efficacy and safety of endoscopic gallbladder drainage in acute cholecystitis: Is it better than percutaneous gallbladder drainage? Gastrointest Endosc 2017;85:76–87 e3.
40. Krishnamoorthi R, Jayaraj M, Thoguluva Chandrasekar V, et al. EUS-guided versus endoscopic transpapillary gallbladder drainage in high-risk surgical patients with acute cholecystitis: a systematic review and meta-analysis. Surg Endosc 2020;34:1904–13.
41. Inoue T, Yoshida M, Suzuki Y, et al. Comparison of the long-term outcomes of EUS-guided gallbladder drainage and endoscopic transpapillary gallbladder

drainage for calculous cholecystitis in poor surgical candidates: a multicenter propensity score-matched analysis. Gastrointest Endosc 2023;98:362–70.

42. Podboy A, Yuan J, Stave CD, et al. Comparison of EUS-guided endoscopic transpapillary and percutaneous gallbladder drainage for acute cholecystitis: a systematic review with network meta-analysis. Gastrointest Endosc 2021;93: 797–804 e1.

Endoscopic Ultrasound-Guided Ablation of Pancreatic Mucinous Cysts

Matthew T. Moyer, MD, MS[a], Andrew Canakis, DO[b],*

KEYWORDS

- EUS-guided pancreatic cyst ablation • Pancreatic cyst treatment
- Radio-frequency ablation

KEY POINTS

- Although most pancreatic mucinous (precancerous) cysts are small and low risk, a percentage will grow progressively to evolve into pancreatic cancer following a pathway that is unique from that of the more common Pan-IN ductal adenocarcinoma pathway.
- This cyst-to-cancer pathway may be interruptible in a similar way to that of the colon polyp-to-colon cancer sequence.
- Alcohol-free, EUS-guided, chemoablation has been demonstrated to be a minimally invasive treatment option for the safe and effective treatment of mucinous pancreatic cyst in appropriately selected patients.
- For safe and effective pancreatic cyst ablation, patient selection is key and the use of a specialized team operating in a high volume, multi-disciplinary setting is imperative.
- EUS-guided RFA treatment of solid pancreatic and abdominal lesions is an evolving and promising minimally invasive treatment option. This approach would benefit from prospective developmental studies with standardized definitions of efficacy and adverse events.

INTRODUCTION

Pancreatic cystic lesions (PCLs) are a heterogenous group of neoplasms with varying degrees of biological activity and malignant potential. Identifying and risk stratifying these neoplasms is paramount, as roughly 20% of pancreatic cancers can arise from mucinous lesions.[1] With the widespread use of high-resolution cross-sectional imaging and an aging population, the incidental discovery of PCLs has risen

[a] Division of Gastroenterology and Hepatology, Penn State Cancer Institute, Penn State Milton S. Hershey Medical Center, 500 University Drive, Hershey, PA 17033, USA; [b] Division of Gastroenterology & Hepatology, University of Maryland Medical Center, 22 South Greene Street, Baltimore, MD 21201, USA
* Corresponding author.
E-mail address: acanakis@som.umaryland.edu

Gastrointest Endoscopy Clin N Am 34 (2024) 537–552
https://doi.org/10.1016/j.giec.2024.02.005
1052-5157/24/

dramatically in recent years, with a prevalence ranging from 2.4% to 49.1% in the adult population, which increases with age.[2–5] Differentiating a PCL based on its malignant potential is the key step, and mucinous neoplasms (intraductal papillary mucinous neoplasms (IPMNs) and mucinous cystic neoplasms (MCNs)) carry a risk of malignant potential that is generally proportional to their number of high-risk oncologic features as per guideline criteria.[3,6]

The prevalence of pancreatic cysts continues to climb and the majority of cysts are mucinous (premalignant), and yet the overall risk of malignant progression is low; consequently, clinicians are often faced with the challenge of determining which individuals require further workup. In this context, characterizing the malignant potential of a PCL is important to differentiate the majority of patients who are best served by surveillance from the minority that warrant surgical resection.[3] However, even at high-volume centers, surgical mortality and morbidity rates range from 1% to 5% and 20% to 40%, respectively; consequently, not all patients are candidates for, or willing to undergo major pancreatic suergery.[3,7,8] Additionally, even after surgery, surveillance is required due to the lifelong risk of IPMN recurrence or synchronous cancer.[9,10] On the other hand, radiologic surveillance programs are associated with significant costs and psychological distress while waiting for a potential malignancy to develop without any therapeutic benefit; furthermore, there are no long-term, prospective, data demonstrating a mortality benefit with surveillance. In this context, EUS-guided chemoablation has garnered significant attention as a minimally invasive, therapeutic option for high-risk cysts in patients who are not ideal operative candidates. The implementation of EUS-guided ablation has emerged as an innovative and promising treatment option for appropriately selected mucinous-type pancreatic cysts (**Fig. 1**).

In this article, we review the protective clinical data related to cyst ablation, patient selection factors including indications, relative contraindications, and contraindications, description of the procedure, as well as recommendations for quality assurance, post-ablation follow-up, management of adverse events (AEs), and areas of uncertainty. We will also review competing modalities, such as radiofrequency ablation (RFA), and the evidence that supports this emerging technology.

STUDIES INVOLVING ENDOSCOPIC ULTRASOUND-GUIDED ABLATION

Since 2005, EUS-guided pancreatic cyst ablation has evolved from cyst fine needle aspiration followed by alcohol lavage alone, to alcohol lavage followed by the infusion of paclitaxel, to the most recent approach of aspiration followed by a completely alcohol-free infusion of a chemoablation admixture specifically designed for pancreatic neoplasia (gemcitabine + paclitaxel). **Table 1**.

Endoscopic Ultrasound-Guided Ethanol Ablation

Gan and colleagues reported the first trial using complete cyst aspiration followed by ethanol cyst lavage as an ablative strategy in 2005, followed by the EPIC randomized clinical trial in 2009, and the Gomez and colleagues RCT in 2015.[11–13] Complete cyst resolution ranged from 9% to 35% over a median follow-up of 12 to 40 months; however, this approach was hampered by suboptimal rates of complete ablation and significant rates of AEs. Additionally, the Gomez RCT also reported a treated patient who went on to develop overt pancreatic carcinoma at follow-up.[13]

Endoscopic Ultrasound-Guided Ethanol + Paclitaxel Ablation

To improve the efficacy of ablation, a South Korean prospective study conducted by Oh and colleagues added the step of paclitaxel infusion after the 3 to 5 minutes of

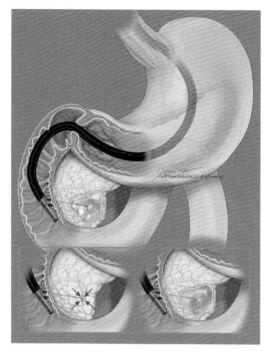

Fig. 1. A step-wise representation of the alcohol-free, EUS-guided, chemoablation process showing the FNA needle carefully introduced into the direct center of the cystic tumor. Following near complete aspiration of the mucinous cystic fluid from all compartments, the chemoablation admixture is then infused, filling the cyst using an equal volume of chemotherapy as cyst fluid originally aspirated. This reconstitutes the cyst to its original size and dimensions. (Image by Devon Stuart, MA, CMI of Devon Medical Art LLC.)

ethanol lavage.[14] As a chemotherapeutic agent, paclitaxel inhibits microtubule assembly and the G2 mitotic phase of replication and is used intravenously in the treatment of a variety of cancers.[15] In an initial cohort of 14 patients, there was a 79% complete resolution rate, and this was followed by prospective studies involving 79 patients reporting complete ablation rates from 50% to 60%, but again with serious adverse event rates of 3% to 10%.[14,16–18] Importantly, long-term outcomes following alcohol lavage + paclitaxel infusion chemoablation were addressed in an investigation by Choi and colleagues who reported results of 164 patients who underwent EUS-guided chemoablation with ethanol followed by paclitaxel.[19] 72% of patients achieved complete ablation and, over a 6-year follow-up period, 98.3% of patients who achieved complete ablation remained in complete remission at follow-up. The authors concluded that this treatment approach is an effective and durable alternative to surgery in appropriately selected patients.

Endoscopic Ultrasound-Guided Alcohol Versus Alcohol-Free Ablation

The inflammatory and toxic nature of ethanol in and around pancreatic tissue surrounding vessels was proposed as a primary driver for AEs in the aforementioned clinical trials.[1] A systematic review of ethanol studies, involving 207 patients, reported a total adverse event rate of 21.7%, with serious AEs occurring in up to 10% of cases, including pancreatitis, peritonitis, and venous thromboembolism.[20] Improving the

Table 1
Prospective studies involving EUS-guided ablation of pancreatic cystic lesions

First Author, Year	Study Design	Ablative Agent	Number of Patients	Average Cyst Diameter (mm)	Complete Resolution	Serious Adverse Event Rates
Gan et al,[11] 2005	Prospective, single center, pilot	5%–80% Ethanol	25	19.4	35%	0%
Dewitt et al,[12] 2009	Prospective, multicenter, randomized double blind	80% ethanol or saline, followed by ethanol lavage 3 months later	42 (25 ethanol and 17 saline)	22.4	33%	Ethanol: 20% abdominal pain, 4% pancreatitis Saline: 12% abdominal pain
Gomez et al,[13] 2016	Prospective, single center, pilot study	80% ETOH	23	27.5	9%	4% pancreatitis, 4% abdominal pain
Oh et al,[14] 2008	Prospective, single center	88%–99% Ethanol followed by paclitaxel infusion	14	25.5	79%	14% abdominal pain, 7% pancreatitis
Oh et al,[18] 2009	Prospective, single center	99% Ethanol followed by paclitaxel infusion	10	29.5	60%	10% abdominal pain
Oh et al,[17] 2011	Prospective, single center	99% Ethanol followed by paclitaxel infusion	47	31.8	62%	2% pancreatitis, 2% abdominal pain
Dewitt et al,[16] 2014	Prospective, single center	100% Ethanol followed by paclitaxel infusion	22	24	50%	13% abdominal pain, 10% pancreatitis
Moyer et al,[46] 2016	Prospective, randomized, single center, pilot study	80% Ethanol or saline then paclitaxel plus gemcitabine	10	29	75% vs 67%	Ethanol 20% pancreatitis Saline: 0%
Moyer et al,[21] 2017	Prospective, randomize, single center	80% Ethanol or saline then paclitaxel plus gemcitabine	39	25	61% vs 67%	Ethanol: 6% (pancreatitis) Saline: 0%

procedural safety of EUS-guided pancreatic cyst ablation was directly addressed in the 2017 ChARM clinical trial.[21] In this randomized, prospective, double-blind trial, 39 individuals with mucinous cysts (mean diameter 2.5 cm, with 72% being unilocular) were randomly assigned to lavage with 80% alcohol or with saline, followed by an infusion of an admixture of paclitaxel + gemcitabine.[21] The primary outcomes were complete resolution at 12 months and adverse events within 30 days of the procedure using standardized definitions recommended by the international position paper on pancreatic cyst ablation.[22] The alcohol-free arm exhibited a 67% complete resolution rate compared to 61% in the alcohol arm showing that alcohol is not needed for effective pancreatic cyst ablation when a chemoablation admixture specially designed for pancreatic neoplasia is used. More importantly, there was a statistically significant difference in adverse events where only the alcohol arm experienced serious (6%) and minor (22%) adverse events showing that when alcohol is removed for the ablation process, adverse events fall significantly. Subsequently, long-term follow-up of this trial showed that 87% of patients who achieved complete ablation at the ChARM 12-month assessment maintained complete ablation 36.5 months later, no treated patients developed high-grade pathology, and 4 partial or non-responders improved to complete ablation at long-term follow-up.[23] **Fig. 2**. This same group is now conducting a larger, prospective, National Institutes of Health funded study using improved techniques.[24]

The continued development of EUS-ablation has transformed this technique into an effective, durable, and safe procedure for pancreatic mucinous cystic lesions, and improvements in procedural techniques, patient selection, and identifying predictors of complete cyst resolution will continue to improve this procedure. The innovation of chemotherapeutic agents revolutionized response rates, and the elimination of alcohol has reduced adverse events. At our center, EUS-guided chemoablation has become a complimentary therapy to major resective surgery, with chemoablation typically preferred for larger, oligolocular cysts that are structurally suitable for chemoablation and surgery typically preferred when the oncologic profile is more suggestive of possible overt malignancy or main pancreatic duct dilation. In terms of costs, EUS-alcohol-free

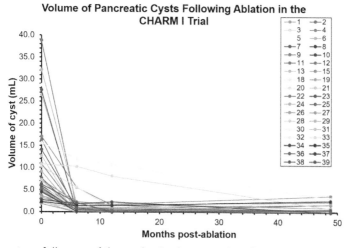

Fig. 2. Long-term follow-up of the randomized, prospective, ChARM trial showing the durability of EUS-guided chemoablation. Shown are the volume calculations from baseline to long-term follow-up after a single EUS-guided chemoablation treatment using an admixture of gemcitabine + paclitaxel.

ablation is markedly lower than pancreatic surgery ($5146 vs $153,215 using *Centers for Medicare & Medicaid Services* allowable charges) which may increase its appeal in appropriately selected cases.[25] Ideally, randomized control studies comparing EUS and surgery are needed and there are no current data proving that EUS-ablation lowers cancer risks; however, evidence does demonstrate efficacy, safety, and long-term durability in appropriately selected patients, and our experience is that it offers a less morbid, yet effective, treatment option that is readily embraced by patients.

INDICATIONS, CONTRAINDICATIONS, AND PATIENT SELECTION FACTORS

Identifying eligible patients who would benefit from EUS-ablation is a critical step in operating an effective and safe pancreatic cyst chemoablation program. Most cysts are small, less than 2 cm and low risk and best managed through surveillance using accepted guidelines.[3] Alternatively, cysts with stigmata of malignancy or multiple high-risk features are best evaluated by a multidisciplinary committee at a high volume center, and surgery is considered if appropriate. For mucinous cysts that exist in the space between these two scenarios, chemoablation can be considered in a multidisciplinary setting. Therefore, obtaining the correct diagnosis of a mucinous cyst (or indeterminate cyst) and the assessment of high-risk features with a high level of certainty is required. This is obtained through the combination of clinical features, radiological imaging, EUS morphologic examination, cyst fluid analysis, cytology, and (if needed) DNA-based testing.[3,26] Additionally, the older and more comorbid a patient is, the more attractive a minimally invasive treatment option is and the impact of comorbidities on a patient's mortality can be objectively estimated using the Charlson Comorbidity scoring system.[27,28]

An international expert panel and investigators at Indiana University and Penn State Health have outlined indications, contraindications, and relative contraindications for determining which pancreatic cysts are appropriate for chemoablation.[1,22] **Table 2.**

Table 2 Indications, contraindications and relative contraindications for pancreatic cyst ablation	
Indications	• Previously identified pancreatic cysts 2-6 cm in diameter consistent with mucinous-type cysts as per guidelines, including indeterminate type cysts. • Patient should have a reasonable 3–5 y life expectancy in order to benefit from treating a precancerous lesion.
Contraindications	• Inability to safely undergo sedation for a 30–60 min endoscopic procedure. • Signs of malignancy or cytology suspicious for malignancy. • Lesions consistent with a benign cyst (no premalignant potential) by clinical, radiographic, cytologic, and chemical analysis (ex. pseudocyst, simple cyst, serous cystadenoma).
Relative contraindications:	• Cysts with the following high-risk features: Main pancreatic duct dilation >5 mm; epithelial-type mural nodules >3 mm; significantly elevated CA 19–9, pathologically thick walls or septations >3 mm; signs of common bile duct or pancreatic duct obstruction; pathologic lymphadenopathy associated with the cyst. • Septated cysts with >4 non-communicating individual compartments.

Moyer, Matthew T and Sundeep Lakhtakia. EUS-Guided Pancreatic Cyst Chemoablation, EUS-Guided Radiofrequency Ablation, and EUS-Guided Fine-Needle Injection. In: Endosonography. 5th ed. Elsevier; 2022:345-355.

Ideally, the cyst should be 2 to 6 cm in maximum diameter with less than 6 locules, since each chamber will have to be individually aspirated dry and infused with the same volume of ablation agent to be effective. Smaller cysts (<2 cm) can be technically challenging as the fine needle aspiration occupies 0.8 cc itself, which could interfere with a complete ablative agent exchange.[1] Furthermore, there is a very low rate of malignant progression for IPMNs less than 1.5 cm, in which a long term study following 108 patients over a 5 year period reported one case of malignant transformation.[29] Cysts associated with a main duct dilation of ≥5 mm is a relative contraindication as the pathology within the main duct IPMN is known to be high grade and ablating an otherwise appropriate cyst will not remove the main duct pathology, which typically cannot be treated using this technique. **Fig. 3**.

PROCEDURAL CONSIDERATIONS

Standardizing procedural steps and techniques will maximize the efficacy and efficiency of the procedure and the safe handling of chemoablative agents, which will need to be done using the individual institution's protocol. We recommend that EUS-guided chemoablation be performed by a dedicated "chemoablation team" of interventionist, nurse, pharmacist, and/or technician. In our experience, this significantly improves efficacy, reduces mistakes, and ensures that the chemotherapeutic agents are handled safely through a standardized process. At our center, the correct amount of chemotherapeutic agent is ordered using a standardized order form then, on the day of the procedure, we call the pharmacy to ensure the chemotherapeutic agent is available, and the technician picks up the agent in an appropriate bag which is handled based on institution policies. Preparation of the mixture and the assembly of a higher-pressure infusion set up should be completed before the patient enters the room. Of note, anything that touches chemotherapy must be appropriately discarded in the chemotherapy-approved disposal equipment. When beginning a program, we typically recommend that you refer to your interventional radiology colleagues and see how they perform similar procedures under the respective institution's rules and regulations.

The chemoablation mixture will come from the chemopharmacy in a syringe with a connecter tube tightly secured, and this will typically be mounted with tape onto an infusion gun *with no air in the line*. **Fig. 4** The maximum dose of chemotherapeutic agents (39 mg/ml gemcitabine + 6 mg/ml paclitaxel) mixed together is 25 cc based on prior oncology studies and recommendations from the Food and Drug Administration (FDA), although it should be acknowledged that this admixture is not officially approved by the FDA for this purpose.[30–34] It is important that agents are infused slowly because the plunger or phalanges on the syringe can bend with excessive pressure. It is important to note that the agents should always remain in the syringe and not be mixed with or otherwise exposed in the endoscopy unit, and we recommend that those involved wear gowns, gloves, and eyewear protection. We generally favor a 19-gauge nitinol FNA needle be used in the procedure; however, a 22-gauge needle may be advantageous in select cases such as smaller size, challenging location (ie, uncinate region), or when traversing intervening vasculature. Antibiotics are not routinely used.

Post-Ablation Follow up

Since lesion recurrence is possible and because there remains a risk of synchronous carcinoma, long-term radiographic surveillance is appropriate as long as the patient's age and comorbidities would allow retreatment or surgical intervention. Even following

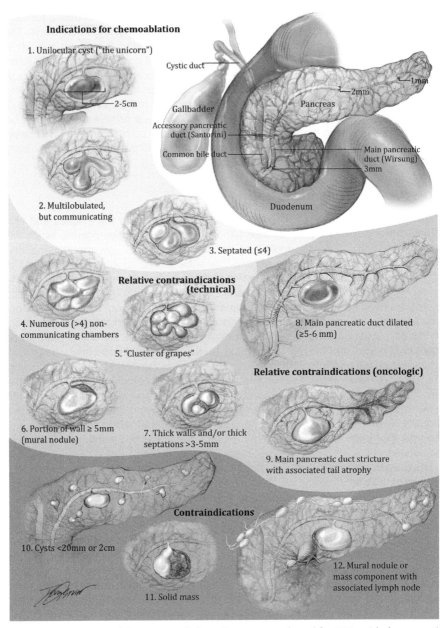

Fig. 3. 10 illustrations of the most typical mucinous cysts referred for EUS-guided pancreatic cyst chemoablation arranged from the most ideal candidates to the least favorable scenarios in progressive order. (Image by Devon Stuart, MA, CMI of Devon Medical Art LLC.)

surgical resection, the risk of pancreatic malignancy remains (ranging from 2% to 4%) and patients require continued radiologic surveillance.[9,10] It is our practice to follow-up an initial ablation treatment with a repeat EUS at 3 months; residual cysts greater than 1.5 cm are retreated.[1] Afterward, an enhanced MRI-MRCP and clinic follow up will occur at 12 months after the first ablation. High risk or atypical situations may

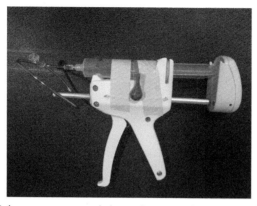

Fig. 4. A typical high-pressure gun and chemotherapy syringe set-up which is required to infuse the viscous ablation cocktail safely and efficiently through the FNA needle and into the tumor. A syringe using higher grade plastic suitable for higher pressure and short braided connector tubing is recommended and as well as PVC-free materials. Additionally, assure that all connections are snug and that no air is in the line prior to infusion. (Image Courtesy Matthew T. Moyer.)

warrant a 6-month follow-up. Cyst resolution is defined by radiological imaging and defined by accepted, standardized criteria where complete, partial, or no response is defined by a ≤ 95%, 94%-75% or less than 75% reduction of the original cyst volume, respectively.[29] **Fig. 5**.

Establishing Cyst Ablation Program

We recommend that patients considered for EUS-guided pancreatic cyst ablation undergo evaluation in the outpatient clinic setting where their clinical, radiographic, and endoscopic characteristics can be reviewed and explained to the patient. Important factors to discuss include the natural history of these tumors, areas of uncertainty, and conventional options of surveillance and/or surgical resection, as appropriate. A detailed informed consent is mandatory, and it is the recommendation of an international white paper that these procedures be performed by interventional endoscopists with training and credentialing in EUS and familiar with interventional EUS procedures as previously described. Additionally, these procedures are best performed in high-volume referral centers in a multidisciplinary setting where gastroenterologists, surgical oncologists, and radiologists are familiar with best practices for pancreatic cysts and can best decide which patients are optimal candidates.[35]

As an emerging treatment modality, there are multiple areas of uncertainty including no clear inclusion on accepted international guidelines, no FDA-approved devices for this procedure, and large-scale studies demonstrating a reduction in the risk of developing adenocarcinoma after mucinous pancreatic cyst ablation are lacking resulting in an area of needed research. This emerging technique represents an exciting treatment option for appropriately selected patients, and further studies are needed to further develop the efficacy, safety, cost effectiveness, and to define which patients are best offered this emerging treatment option.

Endoscopic Ultrasound-Radiofrequency Ablation

EUS-RFA is an alternative technique that utilizes electromagnetic energy and high frequency alternating currents to induce coagulative necrosis within the highly

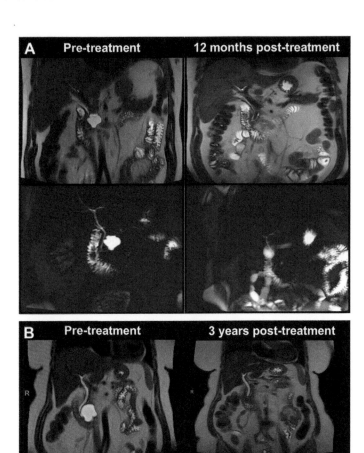

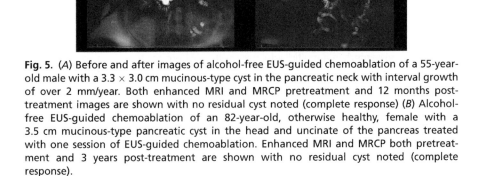

Fig. 5. (A) Before and after images of alcohol-free EUS-guided chemoablation of a 55-year-old male with a 3.3 × 3.0 cm mucinous-type cyst in the pancreatic neck with interval growth of over 2 mm/year. Both enhanced MRI and MRCP pretreatment and 12 months post-treatment images are shown with no residual cyst noted (complete response) (B) Alcohol-free EUS-guided chemoablation of an 82-year-old, otherwise healthy, female with a 3.5 cm mucinous-type pancreatic cyst in the head and uncinate of the pancreas treated with one session of EUS-guided chemoablation. Enhanced MRI and MRCP both pretreatment and 3 years post-treatment are shown with no residual cyst noted (complete response).

thermosensitive pancreatic tissue while also likely triggering an immunostimulatory response.[36,37] The correct level of energy is delivered for variable amounts of time until an electrical impedance of greater than 500 Ω is detected, which indicates that coagulative necrosis of the solid tissue has been achieved from the high-frequency alternating current. Under EUS guidance, an RFA probe can be used directly or through a 19g FNA needle to target the lesion of interest where the probe is passed slowly through the lesion, often in different paths. The usual wattage selected for EUS-RFA varies from 30 to 50 W and if the lesion persists on follow-up imaging, additional sessions of EUS RFA can be considered. **Fig. 6**. As of the time of this writing, the only available EUS-RFA device is the TaeWoong Medical 19g EUSRA Electrode, available in 5, 7, and 10 mm lengths and containing an internal water-cooling system.

In 2015, the first preliminary prospective study in humans involved 6 PCLs (4 MCNs, 1 IPMN, and 1 serous cystadenoma) and 2 pancreatic neuroendocrine tumors (pNETs) where technical success was achieved with two and four patients with PCLs demonstrating complete and partial resolution over 3 to 6 months follow up period.[38] Since then, a small number of prospective studies have demonstrated the safety and feasibility of managing PCLs with RFA (**Table 3**).[39–41] A prospective multicenter study in France involving 17 PCLs (16 IPMNs, 1 MCN) with a mean cyst size of 28 mm found that complete resolution occurred in 47% and 65% by 6 and 12 months, respectively.[40] The delayed response was proposed to be the result of the local and systemic immune activation from intracellular contents released with a subsequent inflammatory response.[40] The same group published long-term follow up data in 15 patients over a mean duration of 42.6 months where complete, partial and failure cyst resolution occurred in 40%, 26.6%, and 33.3%, respectively.[39] A small, prospective, single center, study by Younis and colleagues treated 4 IPMNs with worrisome features and 1 MCN in a non-operative patient and found that complete resolution was achieved in 3 patients while 1 patient exhibited partial resolution.[41] In 2023, the RAFPAN study was published.[42] This retrospective study reported the results of 104 neoplasms (64 pNETs, 23 metastases, and 10 IPMNs with mural nodules) treated in high volume centers in France from 2019 to 2020. Importantly, this study used previously recommended, standardized definitions of safety and efficacy (complete resolution).[22,43,44] 60% of patients achieved a complete tumor response, 32% partial response, and 9% nonresponse.[42] No procedure-related mortality was reported and 22 adverse events were reported, with the proximity of the tumor to the main pancreatic duct of $\leq$1 mm the only independent risk factor for adverse events (OR 4.10, 95% CI 1.02–15.22, P = .04).[42]

Overall, adverse events associated with EUS-RFA for pancreatic cysts have been significant ranging from 0% to 21%, although it has been suggested that these rates decrease with operator experience.[45] Interestingly, the study by Barthet and colleagues changed their procedural protocol after the first two patients experienced acute pancreatitis complicated by infection and a jejunal perforation.[40] In response, the investigators included prophylactic measures with rectal diclofenac, antibiotics,

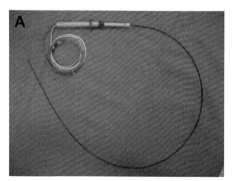
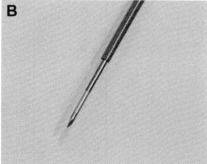

Fig. 6. Example of an "FNA needle (A) type RFA probe (B)". (With permission from STARmed Co., Ltd.)

Table 3
Studies involving endoscopic ultrasound-guided radiofrequency ablation for pancreatic cystic neoplasms

Author, Year	Study Design	Number of Pancreatic Neoplasms[a]	Complete Resolution, n	Partial Resolution, n	Adverse Events, (n)
Pai et al,[38] 2015	Prospective, multicenter	6 (4 MCN, 1 IPMN, 1 microcystic adenoma)	2	4	Mild abdominal pain (2)
Barthet et al,[40] 2019	Prospective, multicenter, open label	17 (16 IPMNS, 1 MCN)	12	1	Acute pancreatitis (1), jejunal perforation (1), main pancreatic ductal stenosis (1)
Younis et al,[41] 2023	Prospective, single center	5 (4 IPMNs, 1 MCN)	3	1	Acute pancreatitis (1), abdominal pain (2)
Napoléon et al,[42] 2023	Retrospective, multicenter	10 IPMNs[b]	5	3	c

[a] Not including neuroendocrine tumors.
[b] With mural nodules.
[c] Study did not specify adverse events for IPMNs.

and aspiration of the cyst before RFA. Additionally, it has been recommended to consider upfront prophylactic endoscopic pancreatic duct stent placement by ERCP (one or 2 days before the scheduled EUS-RFA) if the PD is in close proximity to the target lesion (<4 mm).[42,45]

In general, EUS-RFA may be more ideally suited for solid lesions (such as symptomatic pancreatic neuroendocrine tumors of 2 cm or less) without close proximity to the pancreatic duct and/or common bile duct.[45]

SUMMARY AND FUTURE DIRECTIONS

EUS-guided cyst ablation is emerging as an effective, safe, and durable technique for appropriately selected, mucinous-type, PCLs. Patient selection factors are critical, and as emerging data on long-term outcomes continues, it is likely that this minimally invasive approach will continue toward wider adoption. In this context, understanding the steps to establish a program and team, perform the procedure, handle the chemoablative agents, and use an ongoing quality assurance program is paramount. Working through a multi-disciplinary approach under the umbrella of shared decision-making with the patient will enhance value and outcomes, and where this procedure fits into current guidelines, there should be an ongoing discussion based on efficacy, safety, patient satisfaction, and costs. RFA of solid pancreatic lesions, principally pNETs, is an emerging and promising treatment option when offered as part of a multi-disciplinary program; however, this approach would clearly benefit from prospective trials using standardized definitions of efficacy and safety.

CLINICS CARE POINTS

- Most mucinous pancreatic cyst are low risk and best followed by guideline driven surveillance; conversely, pancreatic cysts with multiple high-risk features or stigmata of malignancy should be evaluated by a multidisciplinary committee at a high-volume center and surgery considered as appropriate. For mucinous cysts between these two situations, alcohol-free EUS-guided chemoablation has emerged as an effective, safe, durable and minimally invasive treatment option in appropriately selected patients.

- EUS-guided pancreatic cyst chemoablation requires careful patient selection, a standardized process, a specialized team, and standardized follow-up. As a result, it is more of a program than a procedure.

- EUS-guided ablation of solid tumors, such as with RFA, is a promising and emerging procedure and would benefit from prospective trials, standardized definitions of efficacy and safety, as well as a multidisciplinary approach.

DISCLOSURE

Drs M.T. Moyer and A. Canakis declare no relevant funding for this work or financial relationship.

REFERENCES

1. Moyer MT, Maranki JL, DeWitt JM. EUS-Guided Pancreatic Cyst Ablation: a Clinical and Technical Review. Curr Gastroenterol Rep 2019;21(5):19.
2. de Jong K, Nio CY, Hermans JJ, et al. High prevalence of pancreatic cysts detected by screening magnetic resonance imaging examinations. Clin Gastroenterol Hepatol Off Clin Pract J Am Gastroenterol Assoc 2010;8(9):806–11.

3. Elta GH, Enestvedt BK, Sauer BG, et al. ACG Clinical Guideline: Diagnosis and Management of Pancreatic Cysts. Am J Gastroenterol 2018;113(4):464–79.
4. Moris M, Bridges MD, Pooley RA, et al. Association Between Advances in High-Resolution Cross-Section Imaging Technologies and Increase in Prevalence of Pancreatic Cysts From 2005 to 2014. Clin Gastroenterol Hepatol Off Clin Pract J Am Gastroenterol Assoc 2016;14(4):585–93.e3.
5. Kromrey ML, Bülow R, Hübner J, et al. Prospective study on the incidence, prevalence and 5-year pancreatic-related mortality of pancreatic cysts in a population-based study. Gut 2018;67(1):138–45.
6. Tanaka M, Fernández-Del Castillo C, Kamisawa T, et al. Revisions of international consensus Fukuoka guidelines for the management of IPMN of the pancreas. Pancreatol Off J Int Assoc Pancreatol IAP Al 2017;17(5):738–53.
7. Scheiman JM, Hwang JH, Moayyedi P. American Gastroenterological Association Technical Review on the Diagnosis and Management of Asymptomatic Neoplastic Pancreatic Cysts. Gastroenterology 2015;148(4):824–48.e22.
8. Vege SS, Ziring B, Jain R, et al. Clinical Guidelines Committee, American Gastroenterology Association. American gastroenterological association institute guideline on the diagnosis and management of asymptomatic neoplastic pancreatic cysts. Gastroenterology 2015;148(4):819–22 [quize: 12–3].
9. Maguchi H, Tanno S, Mizuno N, et al. Natural history of branch duct intraductal papillary mucinous neoplasms of the pancreas: a multicenter study in Japan. Pancreas 2011;40(3):364–70.
10. Tanno S, Nakano Y, Koizumi K, et al. Pancreatic ductal adenocarcinomas in long-term follow-up patients with branch duct intraductal papillary mucinous neoplasms. Pancreas 2010;39(1):36–40.
11. Gan SI, Thompson CC, Lauwers GY, et al. Ethanol lavage of pancreatic cystic lesions: initial pilot study. Gastrointest Endosc 2005;61(6):746–52.
12. DeWitt J, McGreevy K, Schmidt CM, et al. EUS-guided ethanol versus saline solution lavage for pancreatic cysts: a randomized, double-blind study. Gastrointest Endosc 2009;70(4):710–23.
13. Gómez V, Takahashi N, Levy MJ, et al. EUS-guided ethanol lavage does not reliably ablate pancreatic cystic neoplasms (with video). Gastrointest Endosc 2016; 83(5):914–20.
14. Oh HC, Seo DW, Lee TY, et al. New treatment for cystic tumors of the pancreas: EUS-guided ethanol lavage with paclitaxel injection. Gastrointest Endosc 2008; 67(4):636–42.
15. Wellstein A., Giaccone G., Atkins M.B., et al., Cytotoxic drugs, In: Brunton L.L., Hilal-Dandan R. and Knollmann B.C., Goodman & Gilman's: the Pharmacological Basis of therapeutics, 13th edition, 2017, McGraw-Hill Education, New York, 1167-1202. Available at: accessmedicine.mhmedical.com/content.aspx? aid=1162546947 (Accessed 15 October 2023).
16. DeWitt JM, Al-Haddad M, Sherman S, et al. Alterations in cyst fluid genetics following endoscopic ultrasound-guided pancreatic cyst ablation with ethanol and paclitaxel. Endoscopy 2014;46(6):457–64.
17. Oh HC, Seo DW, Song TJ, et al. Endoscopic ultrasonography-guided ethanol lavage with paclitaxel injection treats patients with pancreatic cysts. Gastroenterology 2011;140(1):172–9.
18. Oh HC, Seo DW, Kim SC, et al. Septated cystic tumors of the pancreas: is it possible to treat them by endoscopic ultrasonography-guided intervention? Scand J Gastroenterol 2009;44(2):242–7.

19. Choi JH, Seo DW, Song TJ, et al. Long-term outcomes after endoscopic ultrasound-guided ablation of pancreatic cysts. Endoscopy 2017;49(9):866–73.

20. DeWitt JM, Arain M, Chang KJ, et al. Interventional Endoscopic Ultrasound: Current Status and Future Directions. Clin Gastroenterol Hepatol 2021;19(1):24–40.

21. Moyer MT, Sharzehi S, Mathew A, et al. The Safety and Efficacy of an Alcohol-Free Pancreatic Cyst Ablation Protocol. Gastroenterology 2017;153(5):1295–303.

22. Teoh AYB, Seo DW, Brugge W, et al. Position statement on EUS-guided ablation of pancreatic cystic neoplasms from an international expert panel. Endosc Int Open 2019;7(9):E1064–77.

23. Lester C, Walsh L, Hartz KM, et al. The Durability of EUS-Guided Chemoablation of Mucinous Pancreatic Cysts: A Long-Term Follow-Up of the CHARM trial. Clin Gastroenterol Hepatol Off Clin Pract J Am Gastroenterol Assoc 2022;20(2): e326–9.

24. CHARM II: Chemotherapy for Ablation and Resolution of Mucinous Pancreatic Cysts - Full Text View - ClinicalTrials.gov. Available at: https://clinicaltrials.gov/ct2/show/NCT03085004. [Accessed 24 June 2023].

25. Medicare Inpatient Hospitals - by Provider and Service - Centers for Medicare & Medicaid Services Data. Available at: https://data.cms.gov/provider-summary-by-type-of-service/medicare-inpatient-hospitals/medicare-inpatient-hospitals-by-provider-and-service. [Accessed 25 June 2023].

26. ASGE Standards of Practice Committee, Muthusamy VR, Chandrasekhara V, et al. The role of endoscopy in the diagnosis and treatment of cystic pancreatic neoplasms. Gastrointest Endosc 2016;84(1):1–9.

27. Sahora K, Ferrone CR, Brugge WR, et al. Effects of Comorbidities on Outcomes of Patients With Intraductal Papillary Mucinous Neoplasms. Clin Gastroenterol Hepatol 2015;13(10):1816–23.

28. Kwok K, Chang J, Duan L, et al. Competing Risks for Mortality in Patients With Asymptomatic Pancreatic Cystic Neoplasms: Implications for Clinical Management. Am J Gastroenterol 2017;112(8):1330–6.

29. Pergolini I, Sahora K, Ferrone CR, et al. Long-term Risk of Pancreatic Malignancy in Patients With Branch Duct Intraductal Papillary Mucinous Neoplasm in a Referral Center. Gastroenterology 2017;153(5):1284–94.e1.

30. DailyMed - GEMCITABINE injection, solution. Available at: https://dailymed.nlm.nih.gov/dailymed/drugInfo.cfm?setid=dc02a23b-3ff9-4441-aa91-8e9e629a7315. [Accessed 15 October 2023].

31. DailyMed - PACLITAXEL injection, solution. Available at: https://dailymed.nlm.nih.gov/dailymed/drugInfo.cfm?setid=30ad282b-def4-4269-8a53-a0485d15557a. [Accessed 15 October 2023].

32. Von Hoff DD, Ramanathan RK, Borad MJ, et al. Gemcitabine plus nab-paclitaxel is an active regimen in patients with advanced pancreatic cancer: a phase I/II trial. J Clin Oncol Off J Am Soc Clin Oncol 2011;29(34):4548–54.

33. Gould N, Sill MW, Mannel RS, et al. A phase I study with an expanded cohort to assess the feasibility of intravenous paclitaxel, intraperitoneal carboplatin and intraperitoneal paclitaxel in patients with untreated ovarian, fallopian tube or primary peritoneal carcinoma: A Gynecologic Oncology Group study. Gynecol Oncol 2012;125(1):54–8.

34. Sugarbaker PH, Stuart OA, Bijelic L. Intraperitoneal Gemcitabine Chemotherapy Treatment for Patients with Resected Pancreatic Cancer: Rationale and Report of Early Data. Int J Surg Oncol 2011;2011:161862.

35. Moyer M.T., Endoscopic Ultrasound (EUS) - Guided Chemoablation of Pancreatic Cysts | February 2024. Available at: https://learn.asge.org/Public/Catalog/Details.

aspx?id=YGfmrtzyy19O8D71NwcZnQ%3d%3d&returnurl=%2fUsers%2fUser
OnlineCourse.aspx%3fLearningActivityID%3dYGfmrtzyy19O8D71NwcZnQ%253d%
253d. Accessed March 7, 2024.

36. Canakis A, Law R, Baron T. An updated review on ablative treatment of pancreatic cystic lesions. Gastrointest Endosc 2020;91(3):520–6.
37. Haen SP, Pereira PL, Salih HR, et al. More Than Just Tumor Destruction: Immunomodulation by Thermal Ablation of Cancer. Clin Dev Immunol 2011;2011:160250.
38. Pai M, Habib N, Senturk H, et al. Endoscopic ultrasound guided radiofrequency ablation, for pancreatic cystic neoplasms and neuroendocrine tumors. World J Gastrointest Surg 2015;7(4):52–9.
39. Barthet M, Giovannini M, Gasmi M, et al. Long-term outcome after EUS-guided radiofrequency ablation: Prospective results in pancreatic neuroendocrine tumors and pancreatic cystic neoplasms. Endosc Int Open 2021;9(8):E1178–85.
40. Barthet M, Giovannini M, Lesavre N, et al. Endoscopic ultrasound-guided radiofrequency ablation for pancreatic neuroendocrine tumors and pancreatic cystic neoplasms: a prospective multicenter study. Endoscopy 2019;51(9):836–42.
41. Younis F, Ben-Ami Shor D, Lubezky N, et al. Endoscopic ultrasound-guided radiofrequency ablation of premalignant pancreatic-cystic neoplasms and neuroendocrine tumors: prospective study. Eur J Gastroenterol Hepatol 2022;34(11):1111–5.
42. Napoléon B, Lisotti A, Caillol F, et al. Risk factors for EUS-guided radiofrequency ablation adverse events in patients with pancreatic neoplasms: a large national French study (RAFPAN study). Gastrointest Endosc 2023;98(3):392–9.e1.
43. Nass KJ, Zwager LW, van der Vlugt M, et al. Novel classification for adverse events in GI endoscopy: the AGREE classification. Gastrointest Endosc 2022;95(6):1078–85.e8.
44. Banks PA, Bollen TL, Dervenis C, et al. Classification of acute pancreatitis–2012: revision of the Atlanta classification and definitions by international consensus. Gut 2013;62(1):102–11.
45. Moyer MT, Lakhtakia S. EUS-guided pancreatic cyst chemoablation, EUS-guided radiofrequency ablation, and EUS-guided fine-needle injection. In: Varadarajulu S, Fockens P, Hawes RH, editors. *Endosonography*. 5th edition. Philadelphia, PA: Elsevier; 2022. p. 345–55.
46. Moyer MT, Dye CE, Sharzehi S, et al. Is alcohol required for effective pancreatic cyst ablation? The prospective randomized CHARM trial pilot study. Endosc Int Open 2016;4(5):E603–7.

Endoscopic Drainage of Pancreatic Fluid Collections

Nicholas G. Brown, MD[a,b,c,]*, Amrita Sethi, MD[c]

KEYWORDS

- Pancreatic fluid collections • Interventional EUS • Cystogastrostomy • Pseudocyst
- Walled-off necrosis

KEY POINTS

- Endoscopic ultrasound-directed drainage of pancreatic fluid collections (PFCs) is safe and effective. It is the gold standard for drainage of symptomatic and infected PFCs.
- Patients with infected or symptomatic collections should be considered for endoscopic drainage.
- Four weeks is the historical time frame believed to be necessary for encapsulation of PFCs prior to drainage. However, early drainage (<4 weeks) when clinically necessary and without complete inflammatory wall formation appears safe and effective.
- The use of lumen-apposing metal stents (LAMS) for transmural drainage of PFCs results in shorter procedure duration when compared to the placement of plastic stents. However, LAMS and plastic stents are otherwise similar in efficacy, side effect profile, need for repeat procedures, and overall costs.
- The use of coaxial double-pigtail plastic stents placed through LAMS is safe and may reduce stent occlusion in patients with walled-off necrosis.

 Video content accompanies this article at http://www.giendo.theclinics.com

INTRODUCTION

Development of a pancreatic fluid collection (PFC) is a common late-phase complication of acute and chronic pancreatitis. PFCs as a result of acute pancreatitis are divided into 4 categories: acute peripancreatic fluid collection, acute necrotic fluid collection, pseudocysts, and walled-off necrosis (WON), all of which may be either sterile or infected.[1] Acute peripancreatic fluid collections and pseudocysts occur

[a] Department of Medicine, Columbia University Irving Medical Center, Weill Cornell Medicine, NewYork-Presbyterian/Brooklyn Methodist Hospital, 515 6th Street, Concourse, Brooklyn, NY 11215, USA; [b] Weill Cornell, 1283 York Avenue, New York, NY 10065, USA; [c] Division of Digestive and Liver Disease, Columbia University Irving Medical Center, 630 West 168th Street, P&S 3-401, New York, NY 10032, USA
* Corresponding author.
E-mail address: ngb9002@nyp.org

Gastrointest Endoscopy Clin N Am 34 (2024) 553–575
https://doi.org/10.1016/j.giec.2024.02.008
1052-5157/24/© 2024 Elsevier Inc. All rights reserved.

due to acute interstitial pancreatitis with pseudocyst formation estimated to occur in 5% to 20% of such cases.[2,3] Similarly, acute pancreatic necrosis and WON develop in response to necrotizing pancreatitis with WON occurring in 1% to 9% of all cases of acute pancreatitis.[3,4]

Acute peripancreatic fluid collections and acute necrotic fluid collections are both characterized by unencapsulated peripancreatic free fluid with the main differentiation being the presence of necrotic debris in acute necrotic collections. Both pseudocysts and WON are parallel to the above fluid collections, but they are characterized by a well-defined inflammatory wall, which generally occurs 4 weeks following pancreatic injury **(Table 1)**.[1,3,4]

Chronic pancreatic pseudocysts arise from chronic pancreatitis and result most commonly from upstream ductal blowouts from downstream obstruction by pancreatic duct obstruction related to strictures ± calculi. They are always composed entirely of liquid (pancreatic juice).

PANCREATIC FLUID COLLECTION DRAINAGE: THE IDEAL APPROACH

Previously, when pseudocysts and WON necrosis required therapy, decompression was managed surgically or percutaneously by interventional radiologists. However, there have been paradigm-shifting advancements in therapeutic EUS devices and techniques that have obviated historic, morbid approaches in favor of endoscopic drainage. Beginning in 2010, robust literature has demonstrated reduced complications, morbidity, and mortality utilizing a minimally invasive step-up approach to patients with WON and infected WON in both short-term and long-term cohorts.[5,6] EUS-directed drainage of PFCs is now the initial therapy for these disease states and has been shown in randomized trials to be equally clinically effective, improve patient-centered outcomes and quality of life, reduce health care costs and hospital length of stay.[7–9]

Since the early 2000s, endoscopic and endoscopic ultrasound (EUS)-guided drainage has been successfully performed.[10,11] Traditionally, EUS-guided transmural PFC drainage was accomplished using double-pigtail plastic stents (DPPSs) and was limited to expert centers in the United States due to the technical demands of the procedure. In 2013, the advent of electrocautery-enhanced lumen-apposing metal stents (EC-LAMSs) in the United States generated a profound shift in the modality of PFC drainage. International guidelines are inconsistent regarding the best initial stent type: LAMSs versus DPPSs. A recently revised American Gastroenterology Association guideline recommends the use of LAMSs as the first-line therapy for WON, while the European Society for Gastrointestinal Endoscopy states either method is acceptable.[12,13]

Table 1 Pancreatic fluid collections			
Etiology	PFC	Inflammatory Wall	Necrotic Debris
Interstitial pancreatitis	Acute peripancreatic fluid collection	No	No
	Pseudocyst	Yes, typically ≥4 wk following AP[a]	No
Necrotizing pancreatitis	Acute necrotic fluid collection	No	Yes
	Walled-off necrosis	Yes, typically ≥4 wk following AP[a]	Yes

Abbreviations: AP, acute pancreatitis; PFC, pancreatic fluid collection.
[a] Mature encapsulation may occur prior to 4 wk.

In 2023, The Dutch Pancreatitis Group compared the findings of the AXIOMA trial, a multicenter prospective cohort study to those of the TENSION trial, a randomized multicenter trial, to investigate whether LAMSs improves transluminal WON drainage and decreases the need for endoscopic necrosectomy when compared to DPPSs.[14,15] Though both groups included nasocystic irrigation rather than transluminal stent placement alone, the need for endoscopic necrosectomy, length of hospitalization, costs, and adverse events (AEs), including bleeding, did not differ between LAMSs or DPPSs for patients with infected WON.

Additional attempts to define the optimal endoscopic modality of minimally invasive PFC drainage have been tailored to fluid collection characteristics, including size, type, and location. At 6 months follow-up, the use of LAMS resulted in improved treatment success for PFC and symptom resolution when LAMS was used with selective use of DPPS compared to DPPS alone.[8] This result was maintained for all PFC types (WON and pseudocysts), and the LAMS group had a significantly lower need for surgical rescue after endoscopic therapy. Patients with large necrotic PFCs extending into the pericolic gutters who fail to improve with endoscopic therapy alone may also benefit from dual-modality drainage with endoscopic and percutaneous drain placement.[8,16,17]

Given nearly equivalent efficacy, AEs and costs when compared to traditional PFC drainage utilizing DPPSs, LAMSs placement facilitates PFC access and reduces procedure time. Therefore, LAMSs with or without coaxial plastic stenting is the preferred method of drainage. In patients who fail to improve despite endoscopic attempts with or without percutaneous assistance, surgical management may be necessary.

INDICATIONS FOR AND TIMING OF DRAINAGE

It is imperative to understand which collections warrant drainage and the time frame at which safe decompression of the collection can be performed. The majority of PFCs are asymptomatic and resolve spontaneously, but symptomatic or infected collections require drainage. Common symptoms related to a PFC include uncontrolled abdominal pain, postprandial nausea and vomiting, early satiety, and/or inability to maintain weight (**Table 2**). Those with infected PFCs are frequently critically ill necessitating inpatient and intensive care unit-level care.

Drainage of PFCs should occur at least 4 weeks following the acute pancreatitis episode to allow for the development of a mature, inflammatory wall. Yet, in patients with symptomatic or infected PFCs prior to the 4 week time frame, who have failed medical management, few options exist. In this population, effective endoscopic drainage has been described at a median time from pancreatic injury of 20 and 23 days.[18–20] It is accepted that there should be at least partial wall formation, preferably at the drainage site though a minority of cases have also described fluid without any encapsulation. Attempts should be made to delay as long as possible until a complete, mature wall has formed, but early drainage may be performed if clinically necessary and when conservative management has failed. Drainage until complete encapsulation has occurred remains the standard of care.

LUMEN-APPOSING METAL STENTS

LAMSs are large caliber, dumbbell-shaped, fully covered metal stents developed for transluminal drainage of PFCs introduced with electrocautery-enhanced tip in 2013 (**Fig. 1**). The available LAMSs in the United States are compressed in delivery catheters between 9 Fr and 10.8 Fr, and when deployed, the lumen caliber ranges from 6 to 20 mm with 8 to 15 mm distance between flanges. The flange diameters range from 14 mm to 29 mm (**Table 3**). In their expanded state, the proximal and distal flanges

Table 2
Indications/contraindications for drainage of pancreatic fluid collections

Indications for Drainage of PFC	
Local compression	
	Gut lumen: obstruction/GOO
	Bile duct: Obstructive Jaundice
Infected collection	
Symptomatic	
	Uncontrolled pain
	Weight loss
	Anorexia
	Recurrent pancreatitis
Contraindication	
Large volume ascites	
Unable to tolerate anesthesia	
Pseudoaneurysm[a]	
Coagulopathy	
Underlying malignancy	

Abbreviations: GOO, gastric outlet obstruction; PFC, pancreatic fluid collection.
[a] Relative, care individualized.

unite the inflammatory wall of the cavity and the enteric lumen to create a fistulous connection. The larger diameter of the stent facilitates evacuation of fluid and necrotic contents from the cystic cavity and simplifies endoscopic necrosectomy. As LAMS placement can be performed using a single-step due to the electrocautery-enhanced tip, procedural duration is significantly shorter when compared to DPPSs with varying reports of AEs that are ultimately very similar to traditional drainage techniques.[14,21–24] When LAMSs were introduced, this technology streamlined a process that traditionally required an experienced endoscopic team and, accordingly, permitted expansion of access to PFC drainage.

DOUBLE-PIGTAIL PLASTIC STENTS

PSs were first developed and used in 1978 for relief of malignant biliary obstruction.[25] Since that time, they have been employed for a variety of indications, including drainage of PFCs. There are an assortment of DPPS shapes, diameters, and lengths. They range from 3 Fr to 12 Fr in diameter with lengths up to 18 cm and can be made of polyurethane, polyethylene, and Teflon. The mainstay of PFC drainage with DPPS is performed with the double-pigtail shape to reduce stent migration into and out of the cavity. The lengths and calibers vary based on PFC characteristics and endoscopist preference though 7 Fr stents generally are preferred due to easier maneuverability. Larger caliber DPPSs are often not needed given that the mechanism for PFC drainage is multimodal including through-the-lumen drainage as well as a wicking effect around the DPPSs.

Indefinite placement of PSs should be considered in patients with a PFC in the setting of a disconnected pancreatic duct, who have exhausted endoscopic options and are not fit for surgical management with distal pancreatectomy.[12] This will satisfy the need for long-term drainage and prevent PFC reaccumulation. Placement of a chronic, indwelling drain can only be safely accomplished with PSs.

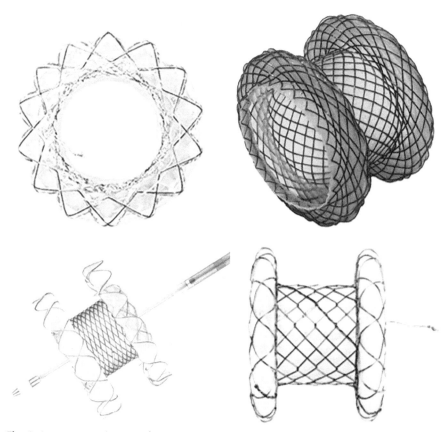

Fig. 1. Lumen-apposing metal stents.

MULTIGATE AND DUAL MODALITY

In a minority of cases, a single site of drainage is inadequate for the resolution of a fluid collection or when there are multiple, noncommunicating collections. In such cases, additional sites of puncture may be necessary for complete drainage, also referred to as multigate drainage.[8,26] This could be considered in collections that are discontinuous or for necrotic collections greater than 12 cm.[27]

Similarly, as mentioned earlier, percutaneous drainage in combination with EUS-directed drainage, dual modality, could be considered in necrotic collections extending into the paracolic gutter and/or noncontinuous collections.[5,8,17] Subsequent dual-site percutaneous necrosectomy can then be performed if necessary.[28]

PANCREATIC DUCT-STENT PLACEMENT

In contrast to a disconnected pancreatic duct, which is a complete duct transection, with pancreatic tissue both upstream and downstream to the duct injury, patients with pancreatic duct disruption may benefit from transpapillary stent placement. Following PFC drainage and stent removal, reaccumulation of fluid may be due to ongoing leak from the upstream portion (toward the pancreatic tail) of the disrupted pancreatic duct. These patients may benefit from transpapillary pancreatic duct stent placement

Table 3 Lumen-apposing metal stents				
	AXIOS (Boston Scientific Corporation)[a]	Nitis-S NAGI (Taewoong Medical)	Niti-S Spaxus (Taewoong Medical)	Microtech Pancreatic Pseudocyst Stent
EC option?	Yes	Yes	Yes	No
Catheter OD	9 Fr, 10.8 Fr	9Fr, 10Fr	10 Fr	10.5 Fr
Lumen diameter	6, 8, 10, 15, and 20 mm	10, 12, 14, and 16 mm	8, 10, and 16 mm	10, 12, 14, and 16 mm
Saddle width	8, 10, and 15 mm	10, 20, and 30 mm	20 mm	15, 20, 25, and 30 mm
Flange diameter	14–29 mm	10, 20, and 30 mm	23–31 mm	10–26 mm

Boston Scientific Corporation-Natick, Mass, USA; Taewoong Medical-Goyang-Si, Gyeonggi-do, South Korea; Microtech- Nanjing, China.
Abbreviation: OD, outer diameter.
[a] AXIOS is the only LAMS commercially available in the United States.

to reduce the pressure gradient across the sphincter of Oddi or provide therapy of any pancreatic duct stenosis that may be the basis of the ongoing ductal leak.[29,30]

NASOCYSTIC IRRIGATION

Traditionally, nasocystic drainage was performed at the time of DPPS PFC drainage. The intent is to allow nasocystic irrigation for enhanced clearance of necrotic debris, prevention of stent occlusion, and reduction in the need for reintervention.[31,32] Using a multigate technique, in which the addition of a separate tract for nasocystic irrigation alone, has also been shown to provide more rapid clinical and radiographic resolution of WON when compared to DPPSs alone.[33]

Though the bulk of the literature for nasocystic irrigation was compiled prior to widespread adoption of LAMSs for necrotic cavities, in keeping with recommendations, it is reasonable to consider the addition of nasocystic irrigation if the patient fails to improve within 48 to 72 hours.[34]

COAXIAL PLASTIC STENT PLACEMENT WITHIN LUMEN-APPOSING METAL STENTS

As mentioned earlier, high rates of bleeding were the initial concern in prior studies using LAMSs, and the intent of placing a DPPS through the LAMS is to reduce bleeding risk by preventing contact of the inner flange on the contralateral wall of the cavity, improve drainage, and reduce migration (**Fig. 2**). The mechanism of bleeding is believed to be the impingement of the distal aspect of the LAMS on the wall of the cavity as it collapses over time.[35–37] Data on reduction of bleeding and reduced cystogastrostomy occlusion remain diverse. A recent small, prospective trial of patients with WON randomized to LAMSs versus LAMSs with DPPSs demonstrated a significant decrease in stent occlusion in the LAMSs plus coaxial DPPSs and an overall reduction in AEs though there was no significant difference in bleeding or stent migration between the 2 groups.[38] To add, larger retrospective cohorts also failed to demonstrate a significant reduction in all AEs with placement of coaxial DPPSs.[39]

Placement of a DPPS through the existing LAMS is technically feasible and low risk. Therefore, our practice is to place a single coaxial DPPS in patients with large-volume necrotic debris or in patients where stent friction at the distal aspect is higher risk for

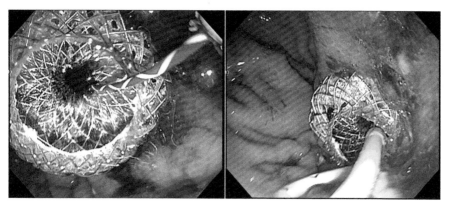

Fig. 2. Coaxial DPPS.

complications, such as bleeding, injury to surrounding organs, or imaging suggesting a highly vascular fluid cavity. For unilocular pseudocysts, our practice is to refrain from placing a DPPS through the LAMS.

NECROSECTOMY

Consideration of interventions must also be given when selecting the appropriate prostheses for drainage. Limited data suggest immediate necrosectomy in the same session following PFC drainage is technically feasible and safe.[40,41] Therefore, selecting a LAMS with a larger caliber (15 or 20 mm lumen) would facilitate access to the cavity and obviate dilation of the stent immediately following placement. The use of DPPSs or smaller caliber LAMSs may also inhibit the use of large and novel devices, such as a powered endoscopic debridement catheter, in this patient population.

DILATION OF LUMEN-APPOSING METAL STENTS POSTPLACEMENT

We do not recommend routine post-LAMS dilation to assist in achieving maximal radial expansion of the stent and for the purpose of stent fixation. In limited studies, there has been evidence of increased bleeding following dilation of a newly placed LAMS.[42,43] However, if same session direct endoscopic necrosectomy is to be performed, then balloon dilation is necessary to allow passage of an endoscope into the cavity.

DEFINING PANCREATIC FLUID COLLECTIONS
Diagnosis

When approaching PFCs, a high-quality cross-sectional imaging is the cornerstone of the noninvasive workup. Prior to considering drainage, cross-sectional imaging is essential. Computed tomography (CT) is the most readily available and widely used initial diagnostic tool due to its short duration, availability, and number of radiologists (and endoscopists) comfortable and experienced in interpretation. We strongly recommend CT be performed with intravenous (IV) contrast to improve diagnostic accuracy and pancreatic parenchymal evaluation. In patients that require PFC drainage, concomittant renal dysfunction and critical illness are common and may prohibit the use of IV contrast. In addition to characterizing the PFC itself, it is importing during imaging review to evaluate the cavity for presence of pseudoaneurysm, intervening vasculature, varices, or prominent vessels at the distal end of the collection that may raise the concern for postprocedural bleeding.

MRI/MRCP with and without IV contrast provides further enhancement of the pancreatic parenchyma. When compared to CT, the superior tissue contrast of MRI enables visualization of the solid necrotic component and can provide more accurate information of the PFC composition as well as improved evaluation of the integrity of the pancreatic duct.[4,44,45] However, MRI/MRCP requires patients to lie still for extended periods and is less than ideal for those who are unable to follow instructions closely during imaging.

Secretin-enhanced MRI/MRCP with contrast may provide improved visualization of the main pancreatic duct to assess for disruption or disconnection.[46,47] MRCP sequences suppress nonfluid signal providing improved visualization of the biliary and pancreatic ductal systems. Secretin is a naturally occurring hormone that stimulates pancreatic bicarbonate secretion by the pancreatic acinar cells. When exogenous secretin is administered, bicarbonate-rich fluid accumulates in the pancreatic duct lumen resulting in increase of the fluid signal and visualization of the pancreatic ducts.

In summary, when high-quality CT with IV contrast provides accurate information and delineation of the PFC, its contents, and the surrounding vasculature, then no further imaging is necessary. If the contents of the cyst are poorly defined, MRI/MRCP with and without contrast provides further insight into the disease process. Lastly, secretin-enhanced MRCP provides the most detailed, noninvasive evaluation of the pancreatic ductal system when pancreatic duct disruption or disconnection is an unanswered concern. We strongly recommend updated imaging be performed near the time of drainage, to reflect the current clinical state.

ANATOMY AND APPROACH

Preprocedure review of imaging (see later discussion) is critical to determine the site most suitable for successful drainage as well as to simplify follow-up access to the collection for stent removal and/or necrosectomy. Imaging review also allows the evaluation for intervening vasculature, pseudoaneurysms, evidence of malignancy as the PFC basis, enteric wall thickness, presence of solid component, and collection size.

A site suitable for reintervention should be considered prior to puncture of the PFC. A cardia or fundus location should be avoided, when possible, with gastric antral and body locations being most preferred given ease of access. When performing multiple-gate drainage, drainage at more than one site, it is recommended to begin with most distal site to avoid unintentional manipulation and displacement of the proximal stent.

ADVERSE EVENTS

Data on AEs remain varied between DPPSs versus LAMSs drainage of PFCs. Potential AEs include bleeding, stent migration or misdeployment, stent obstruction, or buried stent placement. Of these, bleeding is one of the most feared AEs and can originate from the gut lumen wall or from the cavity due to stent erosion on the collapsing cavity wall. The attention to AEs has driven re-evaluation of the optimal stents for drainage, vis-à-vis LAMSs versus DPPSs. In a large, multicenter retrospective study, Fugazza and colleagues reported on the cumulative AE rate of 24.3% in more than 300 patients with fully matured (>4 weeks) pseudocysts and WON.[42] Earlier reports of bleeding were heterogenous when using EC-LAMSs and varied from 0% to 25% though the bleeding in large, recent series is reported at 5.6% to 17%, of which, 1% was classified as severe.[14,23,42,48,49] Bleeding from DPPS placement occurs at similar rate of 22% of cases with no significant difference in time to bleeding or endoscopic or radiographic intervention rates between the 2 methods.[14] Both methods carry similar risks of postprocedure hemorrhage, and bleeding risk alone should not dictate drainage modality. It is important to recognize that bleeding may occur at all phases of PFC drainage early, late, and during removal. Bleeding from the gastric wall can be managed endoscopically in most cases while significantly bleeding from the cyst cavity may require angiographic embolization.

Early removal of LAMSs has been considered an important factor in reducing late AEs from the indwelling metal stent. Four weeks were initially suggested, but recent data suggest the earlier reports of AEs may be less robust.[23,50,51] Follow-up studies have demonstrated both early removal less than 4 weeks (median <3.5 weeks) and late removal greater than 4 weeks (median 7 weeks) is safe with similar rates of AEs, including bleeding at 3.5% and 1.1%, respectively.[49,51,52] Presence of necrosis, the collection size, or timing of removal (4–8 weeks vs > 8 weeks) was also not associated with delayed AEs.

When LAMSs remained indwelling at 12 months, the cumulative risk of bleeding was 6.9%.[53] Early and prompt removal of LAMSs at 4 weeks is based on a single-center experience, and delayed removal has not been clearly associated with AEs. Retrospective data from large datasets support the extension of indwelling LAMSs when clinically indicated.

Risk of LAMS migration either into the cavity or gut lumen has been estimated at 6.6% to 13.6% at 3 months while the migration rate of PSs is approximately 2%.[54] At 12 months, the risk of stent migration increased to 25.5%.[53] The rate of stent misdeployment of LAMSs for PFC drainage occurs in 2.0% of cases, the majority of which can be managed by wire insertion with redeployment of a second LAMS or covered metal stent.[55]

Lastly, the rate of buried LAMS has been estimated at 3.8% and is believed to be related to stent duration, but as previously mentioned, this has not been confirmed by studies of extended LAMS indwell beyond 4 weeks.[42,49,51,56]

PREPROCEDURE PLANNING

All patients should undergo imaging cross-sectional imaging with either CT or MRI; review by the endoscopist is essential to define the anatomy, the location of the PFC, and ensure there is no worrisome vasculature in and around the collection, including pseudoaneurysm.

Electrocautery-enhanced lumen-apposing metal stents

- Collection size: Evaluate for appropriate amount of space from the top of the EUS probe to the furthest end of the cyst to accommodate the chosen LAMS.
- Wall thickness must be equal to or less than the width of the LAMS saddle.

PREPARATION AND PATIENT POSITIONING

When drainage is indicated, the patient must be evaluated for medical fitness for the procedure. It is recommended that active medical conditions be optimized prior to proceeding, which often requires discussion with the anesthesia and medical teams. At the minimum, cross-sectional imaging should be personally reviewed by the endoscopist, and depending on complexity of anatomy and the individual circumstance, it may be necessary to review the case with an experienced radiology colleague or in a multidisciplinary setting.

We recommend following established guidelines for the management of periprocedural antithrombotic medications for high-risk procedures.[34] Antibiotic prophylaxis is generally considered acceptable practice for PFC drainage.[57]

Anesthesia: To minimize the risk of aspiration, our practice is to perform PFC drainage under general anesthesia with endotracheal intubation.

Radiology: Fluoroscopy is recommended, especially when draining PFCs using PSs, although the procedure may be safely and effectively performed without the support of radiographic imaging.[58–60]

Patient positioning: We recommend supine or left lateral position at the discretion of the endoscopist. Interpretation of fluoroscopic images and correlation to coronal cross-sectional imaging may be higher yield with the patient in a supine position.

Informed consent: Detailed informed consent must be provided including risks, benefits, the expected outcomes, and alternative therapies.

PROCEDURAL APPROACH

The following outline describes the step-by-step methods for PFC drainage using the over-the-wire techniques for DPPSs and cold LAMSs (without electrocautery) as well as using electrocautery-enhanced LAMS technique. The aspects of the procedures common to both methods are noted as such.

Endoscopic examination

- Upper endoscopy prior to EUS: Either a standard adult gastroscope or a therapeutic gastroscope can be used for endoscopic evaluation prior to EUS.
- During the endoscopic examination, extrinsic compression of the gut lumen is assessed, as should anatomic features such as diaphragmatic hiatus and presence/absence of masses or varices. Noting location and distanced from incisors will assist in safe positioning of the echoendoscope distal to the diaphragm.

Echoendoscope examination

- Select comfortable endoscope position, when possible. Avoid torque and body contortions.
- Gastric antral and body position is preferred location of PFC drainage, when possible. This position eases re-entry into the PFC cavity during follow-up. Attempts should be made to avoid entering the PFC from a cardia or fundus location.

Wire-guided double-pigtail plastic stent method

1. Using EUS, confirm the collection will accommodate the pigtail of the stent.
2. Identify a comfortable, neutral, and stable puncture site.
3. Lock the endoscope dials and depress the suction button to improve stability.
4. Doppler ultrasound to confirm there is no vasculature within the puncture tract or cavity.
5. Puncture: A 19G fine-needle aspiration (FNA) needle, stylet is removed. If necessary, aspirate and send fluid for desired studies.
6. Tract creation: A 0.025 or 0.035 in long wire (>450 cm) is passed through the needle and coiled within the collection under fluoroscopic and endoscopic guidance. The EUS needle is then withdrawn (**Fig. 3**).
   a. Over the wire, a biliary sphincterotome, cystotome, cannula, needle knife, or biliary dilation balloon with tapered tips ranging from 3.9 to 4.5 Fr is passed over the wire to perform initial tract dilation.
   b. The above device is withdrawn, and the tract is further dilated to 6 or 8 mm over the existing wire to facilitate stent insertion (a 4 mm dilation balloon is sufficient if a cold LAMS is selected).
7. Stent insertion: Over the existing wire, a 7 Fr or a 10 Fr double-pigtail stent 3 to 4 cm in length is deployed. If a second stent is desired (recommend) due to debris or PFC contents, the following options exist:

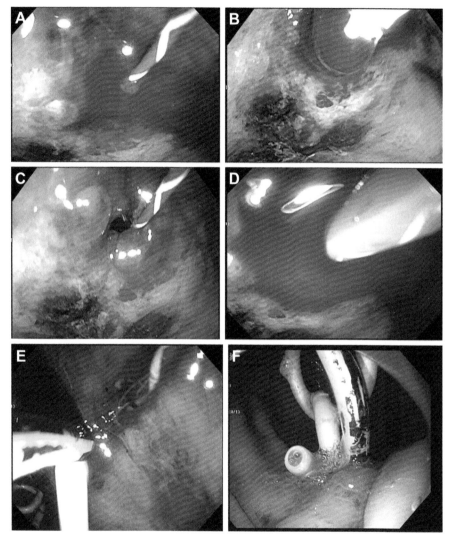

Fig. 3. Stepwise insertion of wire-guided DPPS placement. (*A*) PFC puncture with wire placement. (*B*) Tract dilation with 6 mm balloon. (*C*) Tract following balloon dilation. (*D*) Modified biliary catheter with 2 wires in PFC. (*E*) DPPSs placed over first wire. (*F*) Postprocedure: 2 DPPSs in place.

a. Prior to placing the first PS, a second wire is placed into the cavity alongside the initial wire. The 2 stents are then loaded onto the guidewires and are placed sequentially.
b. The first DPPS is placed, and a guidewire is reinserted alongside the newly placed stent.
c. A modified biliary brush can be used as a double-lumen catheter to insert 2 wires simultaneously. An 8 Fr biliary cytology brush can be modified by completely removing the brush and connecting wire, leaving 2 lumens that can each accommodate a 0.035 in wire. Following tract dilation, the modified catheter is then inserted over the first wire and into the cyst cavity. A second

long (>450 cm) wire is then advanced through the second catheter lumen and coiled in the PFC cavity, as described earlier. The modified catheter is then removed; the desired DPPSs are loaded onto the wires and advanced into the PFC sequentially.[61]

Cold lumen-apposing metal stents (without electrocautery)

8. See steps 1 to 5 above for the "wire-guided plastic stent method"
9. Tract creation: A 0.025 or 0.035 in long wire (>450 cm) is passed through the needle and coiled within the collection under fluoroscopic guidance. The EUS needle is then withdrawn.
    a. Over the wire, a biliary sphincterotome, cystotome, cannula, needle knife or biliary dilation balloon with tapered tips ranging from 3.9 to 4.5 Fr is passed over the wire to perform initial tract dilation.
    b. The above device is withdrawn, and the tract is further dilated to 4 mm over the existing wire to facilitate stent insertion.
10. The LAMS without electrocautery is inserted over the wire and is deployed as described below in "Electrocautery-enhanced lumen-apposing metal stent method" in steps 12 to 17.

Electrocautery-enhanced lumen-apposing metal stent method

1. Using EUS, confirm the collection will accommodate the distal flange of the stent (**Fig. 4**).
2. Prior to puncture, confirm the chosen LAMS can accommodate the gut wall thickness. The enteric wall must be less than or equal to the distance between the flanges of the LAMS.
3. Identify a comfortable, neutral, and stable puncture site.
4. Lock the endoscope dials and depress the suction button to improve stability.
5. Wipe the outside of the hydrophilic LAMS catheter with water before inserting it into the working channel of the echoendoscope to reduce friction during catheter insertion.
6. Use Doppler ultrasound to confirm there is no vasculature within the puncture tract or cavity.
7. When ready to puncture, connect the generator to the LAMS.
    a. Manufacturer generator settings: pure cut mode, 80 to 120 W (400–500 Vp).
8. Unlock the LAMS as one would for an FNA, bring the catheter into view on EUS image. Ensure the foot pedal is ready and in a comfortable position, so that it may be reached without the endoscopist diverting their view from the EUS image.
9. Advance the LAMS catheter in one smooth movement while simultaneously depressing the yellow electrocautery pedal (cutting current) until the catheter has entered the collection as evidenced by boiling of contents (echosonographic "smoke effect") (**Fig. 5**, Video 1).
10. Disconnect cautery to avoid inadvertent injury to the opposite wall of the cavity.
11. The catheter may need to be advanced into the cavity further to ensure adequate space for distal flange deployment.
12. Lock the bottom black lock button on the LAMS device so the catheter is now fixed.
13. Remove the safety lock (yellow tab) to prepare for the deployment of the distal flange.
14. Slowly deploy the distal flange in a smooth, controlled manner until the handle clicks into position. The distal flange deployment should be visualized on the ultrasound image and by fluoroscopy, if used (**Fig. 6**, Video 2).

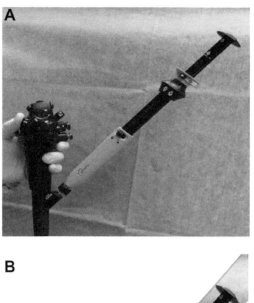

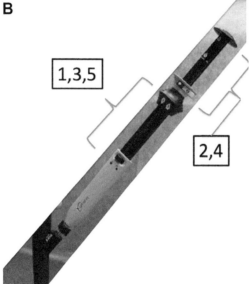

Fig. 4. (*A*) EC-LAMS locked to endoscope working channel. (*B*) Location of different steps on the LAMS handle.

15. Retract the stent until it slightly deforms on the cyst wall/gut lumen junction and lock the device once more (**Fig. 7**, Video 3).
16. Release the top lock and slowly deploy the proximal flange in 1 of 2 methods:
    a. Deploy the proximal flange entirely with the scope channel: rotate the endoscope clockwise and withdraw gently as you advance the LAMS catheter until the proximal flange deploys. Caution must be taken so as to not deploy the flange in the abdominal cavity (**Figs. 8** and **9**, Videos 4 and 5).
    b. Deploy under direct visualization. A black marker on the LAMS catheter should be visualized to demarcate safe deployment of the proximal flange.
17. At this point, once the stent is in proper position, the endoscopist may choose to place a coaxial DPPS through the LAMS (Video 6). If this is intended, it is best to

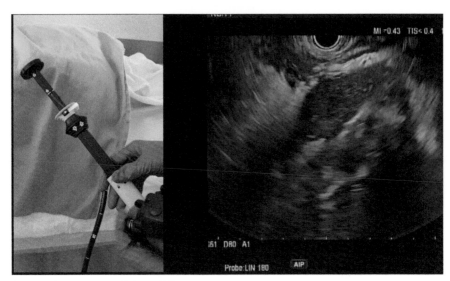

Fig. 5. Advance EC-LAMS into PFC.

preload the LAMS with a 450 cm long guidewire that is advanced into the cavity after LAMS entry and can remain when exchanging off the LAMS delivery system postdeployment.

SPONTANEOUS FISTULA

Occasionally, spontaneous cystogastrostomy or cystoduodenostomy fistulous tracts will have formed and only identified at the time of endoscopy and not previously visualized by noninvasive imaging. Fistula should be suspected if there is air within the

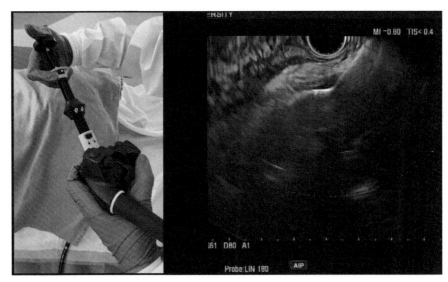

Fig. 6. Deploy the distal flange inside the PFC.

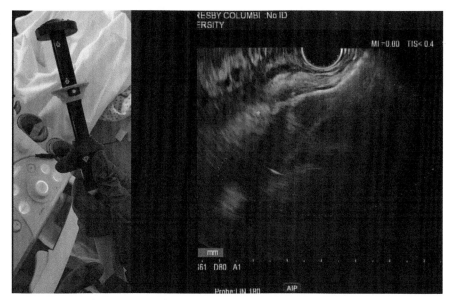

Fig. 7. Create slight tension on the distal flange.

cavity in the absence of prior instrumentation. If identified, we recommend utilizing this existing tract to place a transmural stent rather than creating a second site of entry. The technique mentioned earlier for DPPS placement or LAMS without electrocautery can be used.

PITFALLS
Hand positioning

During deployment of the distal flange into the cavity, as illustrated in step 2 of EC-LAMSs, the hand should be positioned at the top of the handle and the gray button should be withdrawn to "position 2" on the handle until a click is heard and felt (see **Fig. 6**, Video 2). It should neither be released prior to it clicking in position nor the gray "step 2" button be pushed from the bottom of the handle to the top.

Misdeployment

As described above, misdeployment is among the more common LAMS AEs and can occur with either the proximal or the distal flange. This is typically managed with gaining wire access through the newly created fistulous tract into the PFC. The endoscopist can then choose to (1) Gain wire access, remove the failed LAMS, and continue the procedure over the wire; (2) Gain wire access, leave the LAMS in place, and proceed with stent-in-stent technique with either DPPSs or fully covered self-expanding metal stent; or (3) Remove the failed LAMS and repeat attempt at PFC drainage. The appropriate method is individualized.

In cases where a LAMS has been deployed entirely within the PFC cavity, the endoscopist has 2 options. Once wire access is gained, and a new drainage tract is established using the above methods, the endoscopist may either (1) leave the misdeployed LAMS within the PFC and retrieve it during necrosectomy or the next endoscopic procedure or (2) proceed with retrieval after access to the cavity has been gained. However, the latter raises the risk for cystenterostomy stent dislodgement.

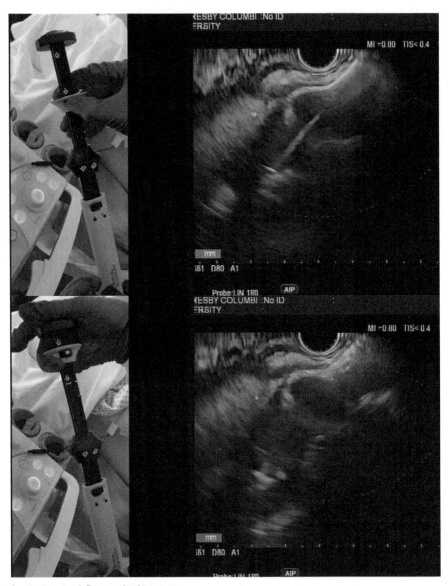

Fig. 8. Proximal flange deployment.

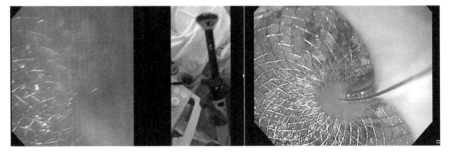

Fig. 9. Deploy the proximal flange (may require advancing the catheter from position 1).

Bleeding

As mentioned earlier, early and delayed bleeding is a known AE of LAMS placement. This is usually managed with tamponade though placement of a fully covered esophageal stent.[62,63] The use of hemostatic spray has also been described to successfully manage bleeding from the margin of the LAMS entrance site.[64]

RECOVERY AND REHABILITATION

Postprocedure recommendations remain heterogenous without well-defined diet or imaging recommendations. Given a slight preponderance for early AEs, our practice is cautious advancement of diet beginning with clear liquids for the first 24 hours postprocedure and advancing as tolerated to a low-residue diet until stent removal.

Cross-sectional imaging should be performed 2 to 4 weeks from PFC drainage and prior to the next planned procedure to guide stent removal, and necrosectomy. For critically ill patients who fail to improve following PFC drainage, repeat imaging in 48 to 72 hours should be performed.[8,26]

Postprocedure antithrombotic medications should be managed according to established guidelines.[34] Patients with infected collections should have antibiotics tailored to available culture data.

There are no recommendations in the literature about use of proton pump inhibitors (PPIs). In patients where PPI use is not high risk, PPI use may be beneficial while transluminal stents are in place.

Follow-up: Strongly recommend a defined method of tracking these patients so they are not lost to follow-up.

MANAGEMENT

The initial insult resulting in pancreatic injury should be addressed and removed, when possible (ie, cholecystectomy, alcohol cessation, and so forth).

As mentioned above, 4 weeks remain for the recommended time frame for stent removal. Although, there is mounting evidence that the endoscopist may have more liberty to delay LAMS removal than previously believed, but only when clinically necessary.

Timing of Double-Pigtail Plastic Stents Removal

Existing data to inform the removal of PSs is lacking. Our institutional approach to timing mirrors that of LAMS for the initial follow-up and necrosectomy. Repeat interventional and subsequent placement of varying lengths of DPPSs for WON is then individualized and repeated until resolution is achieved.

OUTCOMES
Technical Success

- For EC-LAMSs, success ranges from 97% to 100% with no statistical significance found based on fluid collection composition.[8,49,56]
- For DPPSs, technical success ranges from 83% to 99% with no statistically significant difference in technical feasibility between DPPSs and EC-LAMSs.[8,65]

Clinical Success

- No unifying definition of clinical success exists in the literature. It is generally accepted that the resolution of the collection is achieved when the collection size is 2 or less to 3 cm.[8,39]

- For EC-LAMSs, successful resolution of pseudocysts is up to 100% and between 90% and 100% for WON with heterogeneity based on fluid size and characteristics.[8]
- For DPPSs, successful resolution of pseudocysts is up to 98% and 89% in patients with WON.
- A significantly lower incidence of surgical intervention has been identified in some cohorts receiving LAMS for PFC when compared to DPPSs (1.3% vs 7.5%).[8]

SUMMARY

PFCs are a commonly encountered complication of acute and chronic pancreatitis. With the advancement of EUS techniques and devices, EUS-directed drainage for symptomatic or infected PFCs has become the standard of care. LAMSs are increasingly favored by most endoscopists as they are simpler to use, reduce procedure time and enable easier reintervention. Although LAMS and DPPS placement is effective, proper selection is tailored based on unique patient and endoscopist factors. While safety has been repeatedly demonstrated, follow-up care for these patients is critical.

CLINICS CARE POINTS

- When draining collections, greater than 90% of all collections can be managed with a single site of drainage. Additional sites of puncture may be necessary for complete drainage and could be considered for patients with necrotic collections greater than 12 cm or those that are discontinuous.
- The LAMS size should be selected based on the size of collection, the distance from gut lumen to collection, as well as the need for both immediate and delayed necrosectomies.
- LAMS with a coaxial DPPS may decrease stent occlusion and AEs related to cystogastrostomy but has not clearly reduced bleeding or stent migration.
- Removal of LAMS at 4 versus 8 weeks has not been shown to impact AEs, but stent migration rises sharply when evaluated at 1 year.
- Reaccumulation of fluid following LAMS or DPPS removal usually indicates a pancreatic duct leak either upstream to a stricture or disconnected pancreatic duct. The former patient may benefit from endoscopic transpapillary therapy. Secretin-MRCP is often helpful in this setting.
- The chosen LAMS flange diameter and saddle width must fit the collection size and wall thickness.
- Proper hand positioning should be considered to avoid stent misdeployment.
- Rescue devices must be available to address AEs such as bleeding and stent misdeployment.

DISCLOSURE

N.G. Brown: No disclosures. A. Sethi: Consulting-Boston Scientific, Interscope, Olympus, Medtronic; Research-Boston Scientific, ERBE, Fujifilm; Advisory Board-Endosound.

SUPPLEMENTARY DATA

Supplementary data related to this article can be found online at https://doi.org/10.1016/j.giec.2024.02.008.

REFERENCES

1. Banks PA, Bollen TL, Dervenis C, et al. Classification of acute pancreatitis–2012: revision of the Atlanta classification and definitions by international consensus. Gut 2013;62(1):102–11.
2. Singh VK, Bollen TL, Wu BU, et al. An assessment of the severity of interstitial pancreatitis. Clin Gastroenterol Hepatol 2011;9(12):1098–103.
3. Zhao K, Adam SZ, Keswani RN, et al. Acute Pancreatitis: Revised Atlanta Classification and the Role of Cross-Sectional Imaging. AJR Am J Roentgenol 2015; 205(1):W32–41.
4. Thoeni RF. The revised Atlanta classification of acute pancreatitis: its importance for the radiologist and its effect on treatment. Radiology 2012;262(3):751–64.
5. van Santvoort HC, Besselink MG, Bakker OJ, et al. A step-up approach or open necrosectomy for necrotizing pancreatitis. N Engl J Med 2010;362(16):1491–502.
6. Onnekink AM, Boxhoorn L, Timmerhuis HC, et al, Dutch Pancreatitis Study, G. Endoscopic Versus Surgical Step-Up Approach for Infected Necrotizing Pancreatitis (ExTENSION): Long-term Follow-up of a Randomized Trial. Gastroenterology 2022;163(3):712–722 e714.
7. Bang JY, Arnoletti JP, Holt BA, et al. An Endoscopic Transluminal Approach, Compared With Minimally Invasive Surgery, Reduces Complications and Costs for Patients With Necrotizing Pancreatitis. Gastroenterology 2019;156(4): 1027–40, e1023.
8. Bang JY, Wilcox CM, Arnoletti JP, et al. Validation of the Orlando Protocol for endoscopic management of pancreatic fluid collections in the era of lumen-apposing metal stents. Dig Endosc 2022;34(3):612–21.
9. Varadarajulu S, Bang JY, Sutton BS, et al. Equal efficacy of endoscopic and surgical cystogastrostomy for pancreatic pseudocyst drainage in a randomized trial. Gastroenterology 2013;145(3):583–590 e581.
10. Park DH, Lee SS, Moon SH, et al. Endoscopic ultrasound-guided versus conventional transmural drainage for pancreatic pseudocysts: a prospective randomized trial. Endoscopy 2009;41(10):842–8.
11. Varadarajulu S, Christein JD, Tamhane A, et al. Prospective randomized trial comparing EUS and EGD for transmural drainage of pancreatic pseudocysts (with videos). Gastrointest Endosc 2008;68(6):1102–11.
12. Baron TH, DiMaio CJ, Wang AY, et al. American Gastroenterological Association Clinical Practice Update: Management of Pancreatic Necrosis. Gastroenterology 2020;158(1):67–75, e61.
13. Arvanitakis M, Dumonceau JM, Albert J, et al. Endoscopic management of acute necrotizing pancreatitis: European Society of Gastrointestinal Endoscopy (ESGE) evidence-based multidisciplinary guidelines. Endoscopy 2018;50(5):524–46.
14. Boxhoorn L, Verdonk RC, Besselink MG, et al, Dutch Pancreatitis Study, G. Comparison of lumen-apposing metal stents versus double-pigtail plastic stents for infected necrotising pancreatitis. Gut 2023;72(1):66–72.
15. van Brunschot S, van Grinsven J, van Santvoort HC, et al, Dutch Pancreatitis Study, G. Endoscopic or surgical step-up approach for infected necrotising pancreatitis: a multicentre randomised trial. Lancet 2018;391(10115):51–8.
16. Gluck M, Ross A, Irani S, et al. Dual modality drainage for symptomatic walled-off pancreatic necrosis reduces length of hospitalization, radiological procedures, and number of endoscopies compared to standard percutaneous drainage. J Gastrointest Surg 2012;16(2):248–56 [discussion 256-247].

17. Ross AS, Irani S, Gan SI, et al. Dual-modality drainage of infected and symptomatic walled-off pancreatic necrosis: long-term clinical outcomes. Gastrointest Endosc 2014;79(6):929–35.
18. Trikudanathan G, Tawfik P, Amateau SK, et al. Early (<4 Weeks) Versus Standard (>/= 4 Weeks) Endoscopically Centered Step-Up Interventions for Necrotizing Pancreatitis. Am J Gastroenterol 2018;113(10):1550–8.
19. Oblizajek N, Takahashi N, Agayeva S, et al. Outcomes of early endoscopic intervention for pancreatic necrotic collections: a matched case-control study. Gastrointest Endosc 2020;91(6):1303–9.
20. Boxhoorn L, van Dijk SM, van Grinsven J, et al, Dutch Pancreatitis Study, G. Immediate versus Postponed Intervention for Infected Necrotizing Pancreatitis. N Engl J Med 2021;385(15):1372–81.
21. Bang JY, Hasan MK, Navaneethan U, et al. Lumen-apposing metal stents for drainage of pancreatic fluid collections: When and for whom? Dig Endosc 2017;29(1):83–90.
22. Lyu Y, Li T, Wang B, et al. Comparison Between Lumen-Apposing Metal Stents and Plastic Stents in Endoscopic Ultrasound-Guided Drainage of Pancreatic Fluid Collection: A Meta-analysis and Systematic Review. Pancreas 2021;50(4): 571–8.
23. Bang JY, Navaneethan U, Hasan MK, et al. Non-superiority of lumen-apposing metal stents over plastic stents for drainage of walled-off necrosis in a randomised trial. Gut 2019;68(7):1200–9.
24. Bang JY, Hasan M, Navaneethan U, et al. Lumen-apposing metal stents (LAMS) for pancreatic fluid collection (PFC) drainage: may not be business as usual. Gut 2017;66(12):2054–6.
25. Pereiras RV Jr, Rheingold OJ, Huston D, et al. Relief of malignant obstructive jaundice by percutaneous insertion of a permanent prosthesis in the biliary tree. Ann Intern Med 1978;89(5 Pt 1):589.
26. Varadarajulu, S., Fockens, P., & Hawes, R. H. (2023). Endosonography/Edited By Shyam Veradarajulu, MD, President, Digestive Health Institute, Orlando Health, Orlando, Florida, United States, Paul Fockens, MD, PhD, Chair of Gastroenterology & Hepatology, Gastroenterology & Hepatology, Amsterdam UMC, Amsterdam, Natherlands, Robert H. Hawes, MD, Medical director, center for advanced endosopy, Research and education, digestine health institute, Orlando Health, Orlando, Florida, United States (Fifth edition. ed.). Amsterdam: Elsevier.
27. Bang JY, Holt BA, Hawes RH, et al. Outcomes after implementing a tailored endoscopic step-up approach to walled-off necrosis in acute pancreatitis. Br J Surg 2014;101(13):1729–38.
28. Horvath K, Freeny P, Escallon J, et al. Safety and efficacy of video-assisted retroperitoneal debridement for infected pancreatic collections: a multicenter, prospective, single-arm phase 2 study. Arch Surg 2010;145(9):817–25.
29. Chandrasekhara V, Elmunzer BJ, Khashab M, et al. Clinical gastrointestinal endoscopy. Third edition. Philadelphia, PA: Elsevier; 2019.
30. Chen Y, Jiang Y, Qian W, et al. Endoscopic transpapillary drainage in disconnected pancreatic duct syndrome after acute pancreatitis and trauma: long-term outcomes in 31 patients. BMC Gastroenterol 2019;19(1):54.
31. Siddiqui AA, Dewitt JM, Strongin A, et al. Outcomes of EUS-guided drainage of debris-containing pancreatic pseudocysts by using combined endoprosthesis and a nasocystic drain. Gastrointest Endosc 2013;78(4):589–95.

32. van Brunschot S, Bakker OJ, Besselink MG, et al, Dutch Pancreatitis Study, G. Treatment of necrotizing pancreatitis. Clin Gastroenterol Hepatol 2012;10(11): 1190–201.

33. Varadarajulu S, Phadnis MA, Christein JD, et al. Multiple transluminal gateway technique for EUS-guided drainage of symptomatic walled-off pancreatic necrosis. Gastrointest Endosc 2011;74(1):74–80.

34. Committee ASoP, Acosta RD, Abraham NS, et al. The management of antithrombotic agents for patients undergoing GI endoscopy. Gastrointest Endosc 2016; 83(1):3–16.

35. Brimhall B, Han S, Tatman PD, et al. Increased Incidence of Pseudoaneurysm Bleeding With Lumen-Apposing Metal Stents Compared to Double-Pigtail Plastic Stents in Patients With Peripancreatic Fluid Collections. Clin Gastroenterol Hepatol 2018;16(9):1521–8.

36. Stecher SS, Simon P, Friesecke S, et al. Delayed severe bleeding complications after treatment of pancreatic fluid collections with lumen-apposing metal stents. Gut 2017;66(10):1871–2.

37. Lang GD, Fritz C, Bhat T, et al. EUS-guided drainage of peripancreatic fluid collections with lumen-apposing metal stents and plastic double-pigtail stents: comparison of efficacy and adverse event rates. Gastrointest Endosc 2018;87(1): 150–7.

38. Vanek P, Falt P, Vitek P, et al. EUS-guided transluminal drainage using lumen-apposing metal stents with or without coaxial plastic stents for treatment of walled-off necrotizing pancreatitis: a prospective bicentric randomized controlled trial. Gastrointest Endosc 2023;97(6):1070–80.

39. AbiMansour JP, Jaruvongvanich V, Velaga S, et al. Lumen Apposing Metal Stents with or without Coaxial Plastic Stent Placement for the Management of Pancreatic Fluid Collections. Gastrointest Endosc 2023. https://doi.org/10.1016/j.gie.2023.09.005.

40. Albers D, Meining A, Hann A, et al. Direct endoscopic necrosectomy in infected pancreatic necrosis using lumen-apposing metal stents: Early intervention does not compromise outcome. Endosc Int Open 2021;9(3):E490–5.

41. Yan L, Dargan A, Nieto J, et al. Direct endoscopic necrosectomy at the time of transmural stent placement results in earlier resolution of complex walled-off pancreatic necrosis: Results from a large multicenter United States trial. Endosc Ultrasound 2019;8(3):172–9.

42. Fugazza A, Sethi A, Trindade AJ, et al. International multicenter comprehensive analysis of adverse events associated with lumen-apposing metal stent placement for pancreatic fluid collection drainage. Gastrointest Endosc 2020;91(3): 574–83.

43. Mejia Perez LK, Brahmbhatt B, Gomez V. Massive bleeding after EUS-guided walled-off necrosis drainage. VideoGIE 2018;3(1):13–4.

44. Lerch MM. Classifying an unpredictable disease: the revised Atlanta classification of acute pancreatitis. Gut 2013;62(1):2–3.

45. Kamal A, Singh VK, Akshintala VS, et al. CT and MRI assessment of symptomatic organized pancreatic fluid collections and pancreatic duct disruption: an inter-reader variability study using the revised Atlanta classification 2012. Abdom Imag 2015;40(6):1608–16.

46. Swensson J, Zaheer A, Conwell D, et al. Secretin-Enhanced MRCP: How and Why-AJR Expert Panel Narrative Review. AJR Am J Roentgenol 2021;216(5): 1139–49.

47. Manfredi R, Pozzi Mucelli R. Secretin-enhanced MR Imaging of the Pancreas. Radiology 2016;279(1):29–43.
48. Yang D, Perbtani YB, Mramba LK, et al. Safety and rate of delayed adverse events with lumen-apposing metal stents (LAMS) for pancreatic fluid collections: a multicenter study. Endosc Int Open 2018;6(10):E1267–75.
49. Amato A, Tarantino I, Facciorusso A, et al. Real-life multicentre study of lumen-apposing metal stent for EUS-guided drainage of pancreatic fluid collections. Gut 2022;71(6):1050–2.
50. Bang JY, Hawes RH, Varadarajulu S. Lumen-apposing metal stent placement for drainage of pancreatic fluid collections: predictors of adverse events. Gut 2020; 69(8):1379–81.
51. Nayar M, Leeds JS, et al, Uk, Ireland, LC. Lumen-apposing metal stents for drainage of pancreatic fluid collections: does timing of removal matter? Gut 2022;71(5):850–3.
52. Dhir V, Adler DG, Dalal A, et al. Early removal of biflanged metal stents in the management of pancreatic walled-off necrosis: a prospective study. Endoscopy 2018;50(6):597–605.
53. Garcia-Alonso FJ, Sanchez-Ocana R, Penas-Herrero I, et al. Cumulative risks of stent migration and gastrointestinal bleeding in patients with lumen-apposing metal stents. Endoscopy 2018;50(4):386–95.
54. Guzman-Calderon E, Chacaltana A, Diaz R, et al. Head-to-head comparison between endoscopic ultrasound guided lumen apposing metal stent and plastic stents for the treatment of pancreatic fluid collections: A systematic review and meta-analysis. J Hepatobiliary Pancreat Sci 2022;29(2):198–211.
55. Armellini E, Metelli F, Anderloni A, et al. Lumen-apposing-metal stent misdeployment in endoscopic ultrasound-guided drainages: A systematic review focusing on issues and rescue management. World J Gastroenterol 2023;29(21):3341–61.
56. Khan S, Chandran S, Chin J, et al. Drainage of pancreatic fluid collections using a lumen-apposing metal stent with an electrocautery-enhanced delivery system. J Gastroenterol Hepatol 2021;36(12):3395–401.
57. Committee ASoP, Khashab MA, Chithadi KV, et al. Antibiotic prophylaxis for GI endoscopy. Gastrointest Endosc 2015;81(1):81–9.
58. Yoo J, Yan L, Hasan R, et al. Feasibility, safety, and outcomes of a single-step endoscopic ultrasonography-guided drainage of pancreatic fluid collections without fluoroscopy using a novel electrocautery-enhanced lumen-apposing, self-expanding metal stent. Endosc Ultrasound 2017;6(2):131–5.
59. Puri R, Eloubeidi MA, Sud R, et al. Endoscopic ultrasound-guided drainage of pelvic abscess without fluoroscopy guidance. J Gastroenterol Hepatol 2010; 25(8):1416–9.
60. Rana SS, Bhasin DK, Rao C, et al. Non-fluoroscopic endoscopic ultrasound-guided transmural drainage of symptomatic non-bulging walled-off pancreatic necrosis. Dig Endosc 2013;25(1):47–52.
61. Visrodia KH, Baron TH, Mavrogenis G, et al. Use of a double-lumen cytology brush catheter to allow double-guidewire technique for endoscopic interventions. VideoGIE 2020;5(12):688–92.
62. Wang BH, Xie LT, Zhao QY, et al. Balloon dilator controls massive bleeding during endoscopic ultrasound-guided drainage for pancreatic pseudocyst: A case report and review of literature. World J Clin Cases 2018;6(11):459–65.
63. Ichkhanian Y, Runge T, Jovani M, et al. Management of adverse events of EUS-directed transgastric ERCP procedure. VideoGIE 2020;5(6):260–3.

64. Tarantino I, Barresi L, Granata A, et al. Hemospray for arterial hemorrhage following endoscopic ultrasound-guided pseudocyst drainage. Endoscopy 2014;46(Suppl 1):E71. UCTN.
65. Renelus BD, Jamorabo DS, Gurm HK, et al. Comparative outcomes of endoscopic ultrasound-guided cystogastrostomy for peripancreatic fluid collections: a systematic review and meta-analysis. Ther Adv Gastrointest Endosc 2019;12. 2631774519843400.

Printed and bound by CPI Group (UK) Ltd, Croydon, CR0 4YY

08/05/2025

01864724-0003